# 2020 Handbook of
# EMERGENCY
# CARDIOVASCULAR CARE
## for Healthcare Providers

American Heart Association.

**With materials adapted from**

2020 AHA Guidelines for CPR and ECC
2015 AHA Guidelines Update for CPR and ECC
Basic Life Support
Pediatric Advanced Life Support
Neonatal Resuscitation Textbook
Advanced Cardiovascular Life Support
AHA/ACC Guidelines for Management of STEMI
and NSTE-ACS
2019 Update to the 2018 Guidelines for the
Early Management of Acute Ischemic
Stroke: A Guideline for Healthcare
Professionals From the AHA/ASA

**Acknowledgments**

The American Heart Association thanks the following people for their contributions to the development of this handbook: Jose G. Cabañas, MD, MPH; Edward C. Jauch, MD, MS; Sallie Johnson, PharmD, BCPS; Kelly D. Kadlec, MD, MEd; Mary E. McBride, MD, MEd; Elizabeth Sinz, MD, MEd; Jennifer Ashcraft, MSN-Ed, RN; Jeanette Previdi, MPH, RN; Mauricio G. Cohen, MD; Susan Fuchs, MD; Vishal Kapadia, MD; Venu Menon, MD; and the AHA ECC Handbook Project Team.

# Contents

## Basic Life Support

## Advanced Cardiovascular Life Support

## Neonatal Resuscitation

## Pediatric Advanced Life Support

**Note on Medication Doses**

Emergency cardiovascular care is a dynamic science. Advances in treatment and drug therapies occur rapidly. Readers are advised to check for changes in recommended dose, indications, and contraindications in future editions of this handbook and AHA training materials, as well as the package insert product information sheet for each drug.

Clinical condition and pharmacokinetics may require drug dose or interval adjustments. Specific parameters may require monitoring, for example, of creatinine clearance or QT interval. Some medications listed in this handbook may not be available in all countries, and may not be specifically approved by regulatory agencies in some countries for a particular indication.

**Copyright Notice**

To find out about any updates or corrections to this text, visit **www.heart.org/courseupdates.**

# Basic Life Support for Healthcare Providers

## Recognition and Activation/CPR and Rescue Breathing/Defibrillation

*The following sequence is intended for a single healthcare provider rescuer. If additional rescuers are available, the first rescuer feels for a pulse and checks for breathing for no more than 10 seconds and starts chest compressions if the pulse is not definitely felt. A second rescuer activates the emergency response system and obtains an automated external defibrillator (AED), and a third rescuer opens the airway and provides ventilation. If additional trained rescuers are available, they will perform many steps simultaneously.*

*For patients with known or suspected opioid overdose, refer to the Opioid-Associated Emergency for Healthcare Providers Algorithm.*

### Recognition

The victim is not responsive and not breathing or only gasping (ie, not breathing normally). Trained rescuers are encouraged to simultaneously perform some steps (ie, checking for breathing and pulse at the same time) in an effort to reduce time to first compressions and defibrillation.

### Activation

Activate the emergency response system or resuscitation team after finding the victim unresponsive or after identifying respiratory or cardiac arrest, as appropriate to clinical setting or protocol. Retrieve or send someone to retrieve the AED and emergency equipment.

### Pulse Check

Check for a pulse for no more than 10 seconds (carotid in adult; carotid or femoral in child; brachial in infant).

*If pulse is not felt:* Provide CPR (start with chest compressions and perform cycles of 30 compressions and 2 breaths) until an AED or advanced life support providers arrive. For 2 rescuers, the compression-ventilation ratio for infants and children (to the age of puberty) is 15:2.

- *If pulse is felt but breathing is absent:* Open the airway and provide rescue breathing (1 breath every 6 seconds for adult; 1 breath every 2 to 3 seconds for infant or child). Recheck the pulse about every 2 minutes.
- *If an infant or child has a pulse less than 60/min with signs of poor perfusion:* Begin chest compressions with ventilation. If pulse is <60/min with no signs of poor perfusion, provide rescue breaths at 1 breath every 2 to 3 seconds.

## CPR (C-A-B)

### C. Compressions

Begin CPR with 30 chest compressions. (If 2 rescuers for infant or child, provide 15 compressions.)

### A. Open airway

After chest compressions, open the airway with a head tilt–chin lift or jaw thrust.

### B. Breathing

Give 2 breaths that make the chest rise. Release completely; allow for exhalation between breaths. After 2 breaths, immediately resume chest compressions. Give each breath over 1 second.

## Continue Basic Life Support Until Advanced Providers Arrive

Continue to provide CPR until advanced life support providers take over or the victim begins to breathe, move, or otherwise react.

## Defibrillation

Attach and use an AED as soon as it is available. Minimize interruptions in chest compressions before and after shock. If no shock is needed, and after any shock delivery, immediately resume CPR, starting with chest compressions.

| Component | Adults and Adolescents | Children (Age 1 Year to Puberty) | Infants (Age Less Than 1 Year, Excluding Newborns) |
|---|---|---|---|
| Verifying scene safety | Make sure the environment is safe for rescuers and victim | | |
| Recognizing cardiac arrest | Check for responsiveness<br>No breathing or only gasping (ie, no normal breathing)<br>No definite pulse felt within 10 seconds<br>(Breathing and pulse check can be performed simultaneously in less than 10 seconds) | | |
| Activating emergency response system | **If a mobile device is available, phone emergency services (9-1-1)** | | |
| | **Witnessed collapse**<br>Follow steps for adults and adolescents on the left | If you are alone with no mobile phone, leave the victim to activate the emergency response system and get the AED before beginning CPR<br>Otherwise, send someone and begin CPR immediately; use the AED as soon as it is available | |
| | **Unwitnessed collapse, single rescuer**<br>Give 2 minutes of CPR<br>Leave the victim to activate the emergency response system and get the AED<br>Return to the child or infant and resume CPR; use the AED as soon as it is available | | |
| Compression-ventilation ratio without advanced airway | **1 rescuer**<br>30:2<br>**2 or more rescuers**<br>15:2 | **1 or 2 rescuers**<br>30:2 | |

| | | | |
|---|---|---|---|
| **Compression-ventilation ratio *with advanced airway*** | Continuous compressions at a rate of 100-120/min<br>Give 1 breath every 6 seconds (10 breaths/min) | Continuous compressions at a rate of 100-120/min<br>Give 1 breath every 2-3 seconds (20-30 breaths/min) | |
| **Compression rate** | 100-120/min | | |
| **Compression depth** | At least 2 inches (5 cm)* | At least one third AP diameter of chest<br>Approximately 2 inches (5 cm) | At least one third AP diameter of chest<br>Approximately 1½ inches (4 cm) |
| **Hand placement** | 2 hands on the lower half of the breastbone (sternum) | 2 hands or 1 hand (optional for very small child) on the lower half of the breastbone (sternum) | *1 rescuer*<br>2 fingers or 2 thumbs in the center of the chest, just below the nipple line<br>*2 or more rescuers*<br>2 thumb–encircling hands in the center of the chest, just below the nipple line<br><br>If the rescuer is unable to achieve the recommended depth, it may be reasonable to use the heel of one hand |
| **Chest recoil** | Allow complete recoil of chest after each compression; do not lean on the chest after each compression | | |
| **Minimizing interruptions** | Limit interruptions in chest compressions to 10 seconds or less with a CCF goal of greater than 80% | | |

*Compression depth should be no more than 2.4 inches (6 cm).
Abbreviations: AED, automated external defibrillator; AP, anteroposterior; CCF, chest compression fraction; CPR, cardiopulmonary resuscitation.

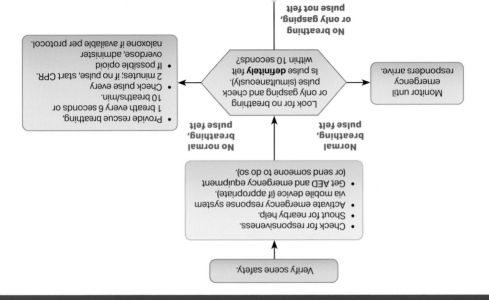

Verify scene safety.

↓

- Check for responsiveness.
- Shout for nearby help.
- Activate emergency response system via mobile device (if appropriate).
- Get AED and emergency equipment (or send someone to do so).

↓

Look for no breathing or only gasping and check pulse (simultaneously). Is pulse **definitely** felt within 10 seconds?

**Normal breathing, pulse felt** →
Monitor until emergency responders arrive.

**No normal breathing, pulse felt** →
- Provide rescue breathing, 1 breath every 6 seconds or 10 breaths/min.
- Check pulse every 2 minutes; if no pulse, start CPR.
- If possible opioid overdose, administer naloxone if available per protocol.

**No breathing or only gasping, pulse not felt**

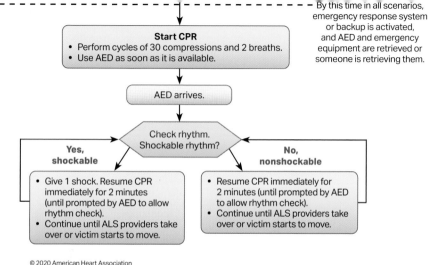

**Start CPR**
- Perform cycles of 30 compressions and 2 breaths.
- Use AED as soon as it is available.

By this time in all scenarios, emergency response system or backup is activated, and AED and emergency equipment are retrieved or someone is retrieving them.

AED arrives.

Check rhythm. Shockable rhythm?

**Yes, shockable**
- Give 1 shock. Resume CPR immediately for 2 minutes (until prompted by AED to allow rhythm check).
- Continue until ALS providers take over or victim starts to move.

**No, nonshockable**
- Resume CPR immediately for 2 minutes (until prompted by AED to allow rhythm check).
- Continue until ALS providers take over or victim starts to move.

© 2020 American Heart Association

Abbreviations: AED, automated external defibrillator; ALS, advanced life support; CPR, cardiopulmonary resuscitation.

## Relief of Foreign-Body Airway Obstruction

| Adults and Adolescents | Children<br>(Age 1 Year to Puberty) | Infants<br>(Age Less Than 1 Year) |
|---|---|---|
| 1. Ask "Are you choking?" If the victim nods yes and cannot talk, severe airway obstruction is present. Take steps immediately to relieve the obstruction. | 1. Ask "Are you choking?" If the victim nods yes and cannot talk, severe airway obstruction is present. Take steps immediately to relieve the obstruction. | 1. If the victim cannot make any sounds or breathe, severe airway obstruction is present. |
| 2. Give abdominal thrusts to a victim who is standing or sitting or chest thrusts for pregnant or obese victims. | 2. Give abdominal thrusts to a victim who is standing or sitting or chest thrusts for obese victims. | 2. Give up to 5 back slaps and up to 5 chest thrusts. |
| 3. Repeat thrusts until effective or the victim becomes unresponsive. | 3. Repeat thrusts until effective or the victim becomes unresponsive. | 3. Repeat step 2 until effective or the victim becomes unresponsive. |

### Victim becomes unresponsive

4. Activate the emergency response system via mobile device (if appropriate) or send someone to do so. After about 2 minutes of CPR, if you are alone with no mobile device, leave the victim to activate the emergency response system (if no one has already done so).

5. Lower the victim to the floor. Begin CPR, starting with chest compressions. Do not check for a pulse.

6. Before you deliver breaths, look into the mouth. If you see a foreign body that can be easily removed, remove it.

7. Continue CPR until advanced providers arrive.

Refer to Basic Life Support course materials for more information about relief of foreign-body airway obstruction.

## BLS Dos and Don'ts of Adult High-Quality CPR

| Rescuers Should | Rescuers Should Not |
|---|---|
| Perform chest compressions at a rate of 100-120/min | Compress at a rate slower than 100/min or faster than 120/min |
| Compress to a depth of at least 2 inches (5 cm) | Compress at a depth of less than 2 inches (5 cm) |
| Allow full recoil after each compression | Lean on the chest between compressions |
| Minimize pauses in compressions | Interrupt compressions for greater than 10 seconds |
| Ventilate adequately (2 breaths after 30 compressions, each breath delivered over 1 second, each causing chest rise) | Provide excessive ventilation (ie, too many breaths or breaths with excessive force) |

Verify scene safety.

- Check for responsiveness.
- Shout for nearby help.
- Activate emergency response system via mobile device (if appropriate).
  - **Alert them about maternal cardiac arrest.**
- Get AED and emergency equipment (or send someone to do so).

**Normal breathing, pulse felt**

**No normal breathing, pulse felt**

Look for no breathing or only gasping and check pulse (simultaneously). Is pulse **definitely** felt within 10 seconds?

- **Roll/wedge victim onto left side.**
- Monitor until emergency responders arrive.

**No breathing or only gasping, pulse not felt**

- Provide rescue breathing, 1 breath every 6 seconds or 10 breaths/min.
- Check pulse every 2 minutes; if no pulse, start CPR.
- If possible opioid overdose, administer naloxone if available per protocol.

### Maternal Cardiac Arrest

Priorities for pregnant women in cardiac arrest include
- Continuation of high-quality CPR with attention to good ventilation
- Lateral uterine displacement to relieve pressure on major vessels in the abdomen to help with blood flow
- Rapid initiation of emergency medical services to direct care and early transport to the appropriate facility

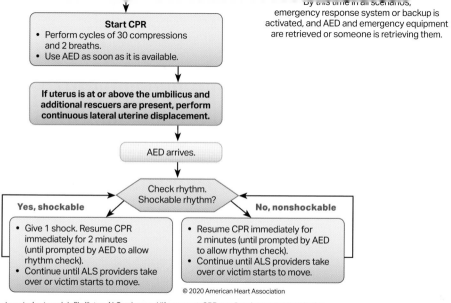

**Start CPR**
- Perform cycles of 30 compressions and 2 breaths.
- Use AED as soon as it is available.

**If uterus is at or above the umbilicus and additional rescuers are present, perform continuous lateral uterine displacement.**

AED arrives.

By this time in all scenarios, emergency response system or backup is activated, and AED and emergency equipment are retrieved or someone is retrieving them.

Check rhythm.
Shockable rhythm?

**Yes, shockable**
- Give 1 shock. Resume CPR immediately for 2 minutes (until prompted by AED to allow rhythm check).
- Continue until ALS providers take over or victim starts to move.

**No, nonshockable**
- Resume CPR immediately for 2 minutes (until prompted by AED to allow rhythm check).
- Continue until ALS providers take over or victim starts to move.

© 2020 American Heart Association

Abbreviations: AED, automated external defibrillator; ALS, advanced life support; CPR, cardiopulmonary resuscitation.

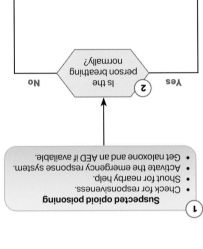

**1**

**Suspected opioid poisoning**

- Check for responsiveness.
- Shout for nearby help.
- Activate the emergency response system.
- Get naloxone and an AED if available.

**2** Is the person breathing normally?

Yes          No

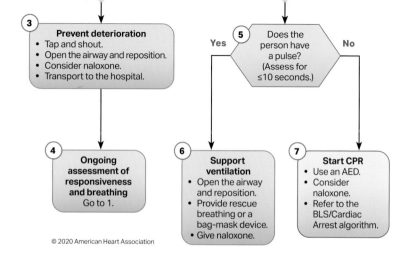

**3** **Prevent deterioration**
- Tap and shout.
- Open the airway and reposition.
- Consider naloxone.
- Transport to the hospital.

**5** Does the person have a pulse? (Assess for ≤10 seconds.)

Yes

No

**4** **Ongoing assessment of responsiveness and breathing**
Go to 1.

**6** **Support ventilation**
- Open the airway and reposition.
- Provide rescue breathing or a bag-mask device.
- Give naloxone.

**7** **Start CPR**
- Use an AED.
- Consider naloxone.
- Refer to the BLS/Cardiac Arrest algorithm.

© 2020 American Heart Association

Abbreviations: AED, automated external defibrillator; BLS, basic life support.

# Team-Based Resuscitation

## Positions for 6-Person High-Performance Teams

This is a suggested team formation. Roles may be adapted to local protocol.

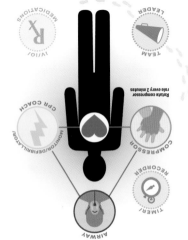

Rotate compressor role every 2 minutes

## Leadership Roles

### Team Leader

- **Every resuscitation team must have a defined leader**
- Assigns roles to team members
- Makes treatment decisions
- Provides feedback to the rest of the team as needed
- Assumes responsibility for roles not defined

### IV/IO/Medications
- An ALS provider role
- Initiates IV/IO access
- Administer medications

### Timer/Recorder
- Records the time of inter-ventions and medications (and announces when these are next due)
- Records the frequency and duration of interruptions in compressions
- Communicates these to the Team Leader (and the rest of the team)

## Resuscitation Triangle Roles

### Compressor
- Assesses the patient
- Performs compressions according to local protocols
- Rotates every 2 minutes or earlier if fatigued

### Monitor/Defibrillator/CPR Coach
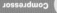
- Brings and operates the AED/monitor/defibrillator and acts as the CPR Coach if designated
- If a monitor is present, places it in position where it can be seen by the Team Leader (and most of the team)

### Airway
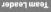
- Opens the airway
- Provides bag-mask ventilation
- Inserts airway adjuncts as appropriate

**The team owns the code. No team member leaves the triangle except to rotate compressors or to protect his or her safety.**

## Key Areas of Focus to Increase Survival Rates

High-performance teams incorporate timing, quality, coordination, and administration of the appropriate procedures during a cardiac arrest. They consider their overall purpose and goals, skills each team member possesses, appropriate motivation and efficacy, as well as appropriate conflict resolution and communication needs. In addition, they measure their performance, evaluate the data, and look for ways to improve performance and implement the revised strategy.

### Timing
- Time to first compression
- Time to first shock
- CCF ideally greater than 80%
- Minimizing preshock pause
- Early EMS response time

### Quality
- Rate, depth, and recoil
- Minimizing interruptions
- Switching compressors
- Avoiding excessive ventilation
- Use of a feedback device

## High-Performance Teams

### Coordination
- Team dynamics: team members working together, proficient in their roles

### Administration
- Leadership
- Measurement
- Continuous quality improvement
- Number of code team members

Abbreviations: CCF, chest compression fraction; EMS, emergency medical services.

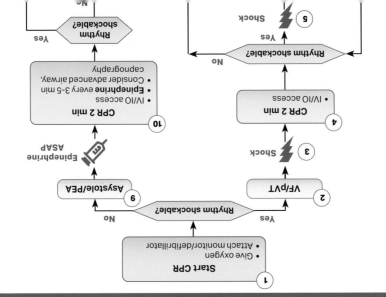

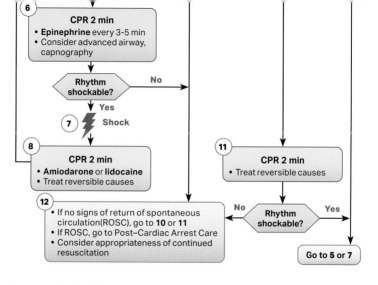

**6** CPR 2 min
- **Epinephrine** every 3-5 min
- Consider advanced airway, capnography

Rhythm shockable? — No →

**Yes**

**7** ⚡ Shock

**8** CPR 2 min
- **Amiodarone** or **lidocaine**
- Treat reversible causes

**11** CPR 2 min
- Treat reversible causes

**12**
- If no signs of return of spontaneous circulation(ROSC), go to **10** or **11**
- If ROSC, go to Post–Cardiac Arrest Care
- Consider appropriateness of continued resuscitation

No ← Rhythm shockable? → Yes

Go to **5** or **7**

Abbreviations: CPR, cardiopulmonary resuscitation; IO, intraosseous; IV, intravenous; PEA, pulseless electrical activity; pVT, pulseless ventricular tachycardia; ROSC, return of spontaneous circulation; VF, ventricular fibrillation.

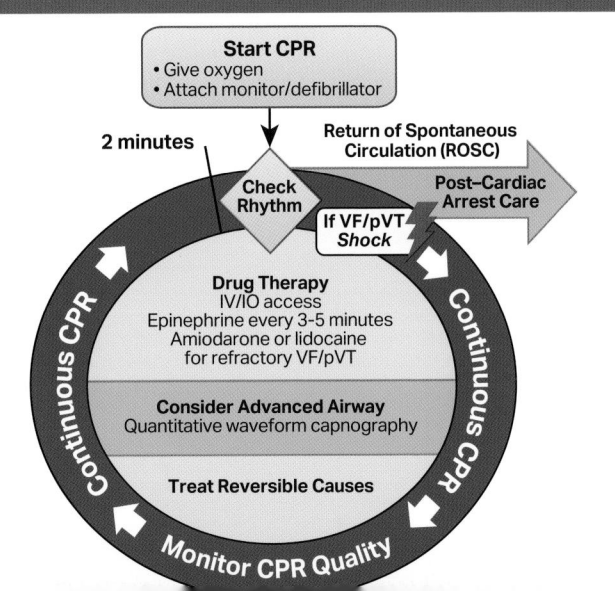

## CPR Quality

- Push hard (at least 2 inches [5 cm]) and fast (100-120/min) and allow complete chest recoil.
- Minimize interruptions in compressions.
- Avoid excessive ventilation.
- Change compressor every 2 minutes, or sooner if fatigued.
- If no advanced airway, 30:2 compression-ventilation ratio.
- Quantitative waveform capnography
  - If $PETCO_2$ is low or decreasing, reassess CPR Quality.

## Shock Energy for Defibrillation

- **Biphasic:** Manufacturer recommendation (eg, initial dose of 120-200 J); if unknown, use maximum available. Second and subsequent doses should be equivalent, and higher doses may be considered.
- **Monophasic:** 360 J

## Drug Therapy

- **Epinephrine IV/IO dose:** 1 mg every 3-5 minutes
- **Amiodarone IV/IO dose:** First dose: 300 mg bolus. Second dose: 150 mg.
- **Lidocaine IV/IO dose:** First dose: 1-1.5 mg/kg. Second dose: 0.5-0.75 mg/kg.

## Advanced Airway

- Endotracheal intubation or supraglottic advanced airway
- Waveform capnography or capnometry to confirm and monitor ET tube placement
- Once advanced airway in place, give 1 breath every 6 seconds (10 breaths/min) with continuous chest compressions

## Return of Spontaneous Circulation (ROSC)

- Pulse and blood pressure
- Abrupt sustained increase in $PETCO_2$ (typically ≥40 mm Hg)
- Spontaneous arterial pressure waves with intra-arterial monitoring

## Reversible Causes

- **H**ypovolemia
- **H**ypoxia
- **H**ydrogen ion (acidosis)
- **H**ypo-/hyperkalemia
- **H**ypothermia
- **T**ension pneumothorax
- **T**amponade, cardiac
- **T**oxins
- **T**hrombosis, pulmonary
- **T**hrombosis, coronary

Abbreviations: CPR, cardiopulmonary resuscitation; ET, endotracheal; IO, intraosseous; IV, intravenous; pVT, pulseless ventricular tachycardia; ROSC, return of spontaneous circulation; VF, ventricular fibrillation.

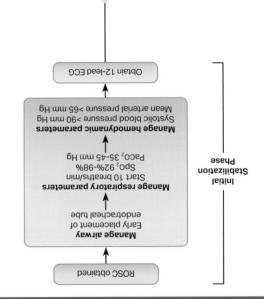

**ROSC obtained**

## Initial Stabilization Phase

**Manage airway**
Early placement of endotracheal tube

**Manage respiratory parameters**
Start 10 breaths/min
Spo₂ 92%-98%
Paco₂ 35-45 mm Hg

**Manage hemodynamic parameters**
Systolic blood pressure >90 mm Hg
Mean arterial pressure >65 mm Hg

**Obtain 12-lead ECG**

---

## Initial Stabilization Phase

Resuscitation is ongoing during the post-ROSC phase, and many of these activities can occur concurrently. However, if prioritization is necessary, follow these steps:

- **Airway management:** Waveform capnography or capnometry to confirm and monitor endotracheal tube placement
- **Manage respiratory parameters:** Titrate Fio₂ for Spo₂ 92%-98%; start at 10 breaths/min; titrate to Paco₂ of 35-45 mm Hg
- **Manage hemodynamic parameters:** Administer crystalloid and/or vasopressor or inotrope for goal systolic blood pressure >90 mm Hg or mean arterial pressure >65 mm Hg

## Continued Management and Additional Emergent Activities

These evaluations should be done concurrently so that decisions on targeted temperature management (TTM) receive high priority as cardiac interventions.

- **Emergent cardiac intervention:** Early evaluation of 12-lead electrocardiogram (ECG); consider hemodynamics for decision on cardiac intervention
- **TTM:** If patient is not following commands, start TTM as soon as possible; begin at 32-36°C for 24 hours by using a cooling device with feedback loop

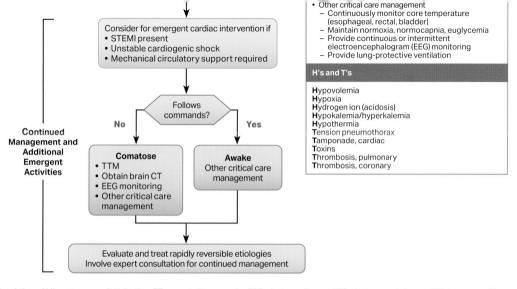

Consider for emergent cardiac intervention if
- STEMI present
- Unstable cardiogenic shock
- Mechanical circulatory support required

- Other critical care management
  - Continuously monitor core temperature (esophageal, rectal, bladder)
  - Maintain normoxia, normocapnia, euglycemia
  - Provide continuous or intermittent electroencephalogram (EEG) monitoring
  - Provide lung-protective ventilation

**H's and T's**

**H**ypovolemia
**H**ypoxia
**H**ydrogen ion (acidosis)
**H**ypokalemia/hyperkalemia
**H**ypothermia
**T**ension pneumothorax
**T**amponade, cardiac
**T**oxins
**T**hrombosis, pulmonary
**T**hrombosis, coronary

**Follows commands?**

No      Yes

**Continued Management and Additional Emergent Activities**

**Comatose**
- TTM
- Obtain brain CT
- EEG monitoring
- Other critical care management

**Awake**
Other critical care management

Evaluate and treat rapidly reversible etiologies
Involve expert consultation for continued management

Abbreviations: AMI, acute myocardial infarction; CT, computed tomography; ECG, electrocardiogram; EEG, electroencephalogram; IO, intraosseous; IV, intravenous; ROSC, return of spontaneous circulation; STEMI, ST-segment elevation myocardial infarction; TTM, targeted temperature management.

Assess appropriateness for clinical condition.
Heart rate typically <50/min if bradyarrhythmia.

**Identify and treat underlying cause**

- Maintain patent airway; assist breathing as necessary
- Oxygen (if hypoxemic)
- Cardiac monitor to identify rhythm; monitor blood pressure and oximetry
- IV access
- 12-Lead ECG if available; don't delay therapy
- Consider possible hypoxic and toxicologic causes

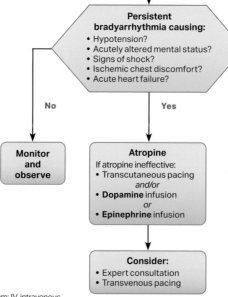

**Doses/Details**

**Atropine IV dose:** First dose: 1 mg bolus. Repeat every 3-5 minutes. Maximum: 3 mg.

**Dopamine IV infusion:** Usual infusion rate is 5-20 mcg/kg per minute. Titrate to patient response; taper slowly.

**Epinephrine IV infusion:** 2-10 mcg per minute infusion. Titrate to patient response.

**Causes:**
- Myocardial ischemia/infarction
- Drugs/toxicologic (eg, calcium channel blockers, beta-blockers, digoxin)
- Hypoxia
- Electrolyte abnormality (eg, hyperkalemia)

Abbreviations: ECG, electrocardiogram; IV, intravenous.

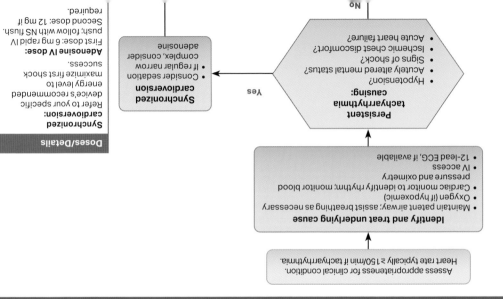

Assess appropriateness for clinical condition.
Heart rate typically ≥ 150/min if tachyarrhythmia.

**Identify and treat underlying cause**

- Maintain patent airway; assist breathing as necessary
- Oxygen (if hypoxemic)
- Cardiac monitor to identify rhythm; monitor blood pressure and oximetry
- IV access
- 12-lead ECG, if available

**Persistent tachyarrhythmia causing:**

- Hypotension?
- Acutely altered mental status?
- Signs of shock?
- Ischemic chest discomfort?
- Acute heart failure?

**No**

**Yes**

**Synchronized cardioversion**

- Consider sedation
- If regular narrow complex, consider adenosine

**Doses/Details**

**Synchronized cardioversion:**
Refer to your specific device's recommended energy level to maximize first shock success.

**Adenosine IV dose:**
First dose: 6 mg rapid IV push; follow with NS flush.
Second dose: 12 mg if required.

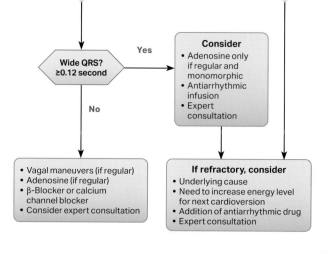

**Antiarrhythmic Infusions for Stable Wide-QRS Tachycardia**

**Procainamide IV dose:**
20-50 mg/min until arrhythmia suppressed, hypotension ensues, QRS duration increases >50%, or maximum dose 17 mg/kg given. Maintenance infusion: 1-4 mg/min. Avoid if prolonged QT or CHF.

**Amiodarone IV dose:**
First dose: 150 mg over 10 minutes. Repeat as needed if VT recurs. Follow by maintenance infusion of 1 mg/min for first 6 hours.

**Sotalol IV dose:**
100 mg (1.5 mg/kg) over 5 minutes. Avoid if prolonged QT.

---

**Wide QRS?**
≥0.12 second

Yes →

**Consider**
- Adenosine only if regular and monomorphic
- Antiarrhythmic infusion
- Expert consultation

No ↓

- Vagal maneuvers (if regular)
- Adenosine (if regular)
- β-Blocker or calcium channel blocker
- Consider expert consultation

**If refractory, consider**
- Underlying cause
- Need to increase energy level for next cardioversion
- Addition of antiarrhythmic drug
- Expert consultation

Abbreviations: CHF, congestive heart failure; ECG, electrocardiogram; IV, intravenous; NS, normal saline; VT, ventricular tachycardia.

Rhythm strips A and B demonstrate the requirement to evaluate the QT interval in light of the heart rate. Strip C depicts an ECG from a patient with a prolonged QT interval.

- *Strip A:* A bradycardic rhythm of 57/min has a QT interval of 0.4 second, which is less than the upper limit of normal for a rate of 57 (0.41 second for a man and 0.45 second for a woman), and a QT/R-R ratio of 38% (<40%).

- *Strip B:* A faster rate of 78/min has a shorter measured QT interval of 0.24 second (faster-shorter/slower-longer), which is less than the upper limit of normal for a rate of 78 (0.35 second for a man and 0.38 second for a woman), and a QT/R-R ratio of 33% (<40%).

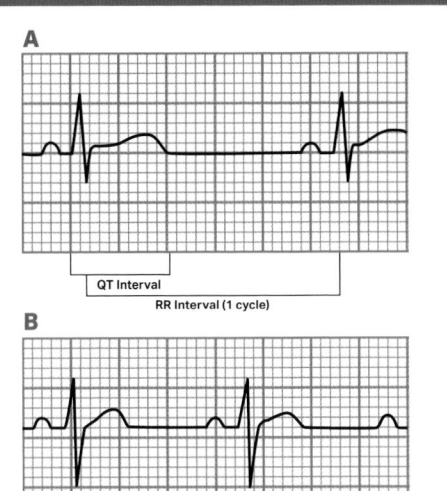

A

QT Interval

RR Interval (1 cycle)

B

QT Interval

*Strip C.* Here the QT interval is prolonged at 0.45 second, exceeding the upper limit of normal for a rate of 80/min (0.34 second for a man and 0.37 second for a woman). The QT/R-R ratio of 59% is considerably above the 40% threshold. This strip is from a patient who took an overdose of a tricyclic antidepressant.

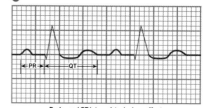

Prolonged QT interval: toxic drug effects

| Parameter | Rhythm strip A | Rhythm strip B | Rhythm strip C |
|---|---|---|---|
| Rate | 57/min | 78/min | 80/min |
| R-R interval (cardiac cycle time) | 1.04 seconds (26 × 1-mm boxes) | 0.72 second (18 × 1-mm boxes) | 0.76 second (19 × 1-mm boxes) |
| QT interval, measured | 0.4 second (10 × 1-mm boxes) | 0.24 second (6 × 1-mm boxes) | 0.45 second (11 × 1-mm boxes) |
| QT$_c$ interval: QT interval corrected for heart rate (upper limit of normal QT interval range for a man or a woman from table on next page) | 0.41 second (man) 0.45 second (woman) | 0.35 second (man) 0.38 second (woman) | 0.34 second (man) 0.37 second (woman) |
| QT/R-R ratio: QT interval divided by R-R interval | 38% (0.4/1.04 = 0.384) | 33% (0.24/0.72 = 0.333) | 59% (0.45/0.76 = 0.592) |

From Cummins RO, Graves JR. *ACLS Scenarios: Core Concepts for Case-Based Learning.* Mosby Lifeline; 1996. Figures modified with permission from Elsevier.

# Maximum QT Interval (Upper Limits of Normal) for Men and Women Based on Heart Rate

Note the relationship between decreasing heart rate and increasing maximum QT interval. For normal heart range of 60 to 100/min, the maximum QT intervals for men and women are less than one half the R-R interval. Most people estimate QT and R-R intervals by counting the number of 1-mm boxes and then multiplying by 0.04 second.

| Heart rate (per minute) (note decreasing) | R-R interval or "cycle time" (sec) (note increasing) | Upper limits of normal QT interval in men (sec) (note increasing) | Upper limits of normal QT interval in women (sec) (note increasing) |
|---|---|---|---|
| 150 | 0.4 | 0.25 | 0.28 |
| 136 | 0.44 | 0.26 | 0.29 |
| 125 | 0.48 | 0.28 | 0.3 |
| 115 | 0.52 | 0.29 | 0.32 |
| 107 | 0.56 | 0.3 | 0.33 |
| 100 | 0.6 | 0.31 | 0.34 |
| 93 | 0.64 | 0.32 | 0.35 |
| 88 | 0.68 | 0.33 | 0.36 |
| 78 | 0.72 | 0.35 | 0.38 |

(continued)

| 75 | 0.8 | 0.36 | 0.39 |
|----|-----|------|------|
| 71 | 0.84 | 0.37 | 0.4 |
| 68 | 0.88 | 0.38 | 0.41 |
| 65 | 0.92 | 0.38 | 0.42 |
| 62 | 0.96 | 0.39 | 0.43 |
| 60 | 1 | 0.4 | 0.44 |
| 57 | 1.04 | 0.41 | 0.45 |
| 52 | 1.08 | 0.42 | 0.47 |
| 50 | 1.2 | 0.44 | 0.48 |

From Cummins RO, Graves JR. *ACLS Scenarios: Core Concepts for Case-Based Learning.* St Louis, MO: Mosby Lifeline; 1996. Copyright Elsevier.

# Electrical Cardioversion Algorithm

**Tachycardia**
With serious signs and symptoms related to the tachycardia

↓

If ventricular rate is < 150/min, prepare for **immediate cardioversion.** May give brief trial of medications based on specific arrhythmias. Immediate cardioversion is generally not needed if heart rate is ≤150/min.

↓

Have available at beside
- Oxygen saturation monitor
- Suction device
- IV line
- Intubation equipment

## Steps for Adult Defibrillation and Cardioversion Using Manual Defibrillators (Monophasic or Biphasic)

*Assess the rhythm. If ventricular fibrillation (VF) or pulseless ventricular tachycardia (pVT) is present, continue chest compressions without interruptions during all steps until step 8.*

### Defibrillation (for VF and pVT)

1. Turn on defibrillator. For biphasic defibrillators, use manufacturer-specific energy if known. For monophasic defibrillators, use 360 J. If unknown, select the maximum energy available.

2. Set lead select switch to paddles (or lead I, II, or III if monitor leads are used).

3. Prepare adhesive pads (pads are preferred); if using paddles, apply appropriate conductive gel or paste. Be sure cables are attached to defibrillator.

4. Position defibrillation pads on patient's chest following manufacturer's recommendations. If using paddles, place one paddle on the right anterior chest wall and one in the left axillary position, applying firm pressure (about 15-25 pounds) when ready to deliver shock. If patient has an implanted pacemaker, position the pads/paddles so they are not directly over the device. Be sure that oxygen flow is not directed across the patient's chest.

5. Announce "Charging defibrillator!"

6. Press charge button on apex paddle or defibrillator controls.

7. When the defibrillator is fully charged, state firmly: "I am going to shock on three." "Then count, "I am clear to shock!" (Chest compressions should continue until this announcement.)

8. After confirming all personnel are clear of the patient, press the shock button on the defibrillator or press the 2 paddle discharge buttons simultaneously.

9. Immediately after the shock is delivered, resume CPR, beginning with compressions for 2 minutes, and then recheck rhythm. Interruption of

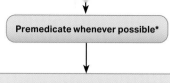

**Premedicate whenever possible***

↓

### *Synchronized cardioversion†‡*

Refer to your specific device's recommended energy level to maximize first shock success.

### Notes

*Effective regimens have included a sedative **(eg, diazepam, midazolam, etomidate, methohexital, propofol)** with or without an analgesic agent **(eg, fentanyl, morphine)**. Many experts recommend anesthesia if service is readily available.

†Note possible need to resynchronize after each cardioversion.

‡If delays in synchronization occur and clinical condition is critical, go immediately to unsynchronized shocks.

## Cardioversion (for tachycardia with a pulse)

*Assess the rhythm. If patient has a pulse but is unstable, proceed with cardioversion.*

**1-4.** Follow steps for defibrillation above (except for energy dose).

**5.** Consider sedation.

**6.** Engage the ***synchronization*** mode by pressing the *sync control* button.

**7.** Look for markers on R waves indicating *sync* mode is operative. If necessary, adjust monitor gain until sync markers occur with each R wave.

**8.** Select appropriate energy level (see Electrical Cardioversion Algorithm on left).

**9.** Announce "Charging defibrillator!"

**10.** Press *charge* button on apex paddle or defibrillator controls.

**11.** When the defibrillator is fully charged, state firmly: "I am going to shock on three." Then count. "I am clear to shock!"

**12.** After confirming all personnel are clear of the patient, press the *discharge* buttons simultaneously on paddles or the *shock* button on the unit; hold paddles in place until shock is delivered.

**13.** Check the monitor. If tachycardia persists, increase the energy and prepare to cardiovert again.

**14.** Reset the ***sync*** mode after each synchronized cardioversion because most defibrillators default back to *unsynchronized* mode. This default allows an immediate shock if the cardioversion produces VF.

| Therapy | Indications/precautions | Adult dosage |
| --- | --- | --- |
| **Cardioversion** (Synchronized)<br><br>• Administered via adhesive defibrillation electrode pads or handheld paddles<br>• Place defibrillator/monitor in synchronized (sync) mode<br>• Sync mode delivers energy concurrent with the QRS | **Indications**<br>• All unstable tachycardias (rate < 150/min) with signs and symptoms related to tachycardia (acutely altered mental status, ischemic chest discomfort, acute heart failure, hypotension, or other signs of shock).<br>• A brief trial of medications is an alternative first step for specific arrhythmias.<br><br>**Precautions/Contraindications**<br>• If patient is unresponsive, go to immediate unsynchronized shocks.<br>• Urgent cardioversion is generally not needed if heart rate is ≤150/min.<br>• Be sure oxygen is not flowing across patient's chest.<br>• Direct flow away from patient's chest and consider temporarily disconnecting bag or ventilation circuit from endotracheal tube during shock delivery.<br>• Reactivation of sync mode is required after each attempted cardioversion (defibrillator/cardioverter defaults to unsynchronized mode).<br>• Prepare to defibrillate immediately if cardioversion causes ventricular fibrillation. | **Technique**<br>• Consider premedicating with sedatives if the patient is conscious.<br>• Engage *sync* mode before each attempt.<br>• Look for sync markers on the R wave.<br>• Clear all personnel from the patient before each shock.<br>• Refer to your specific device's recommended energy level to maximize first shock success.<br>• *Irregular wide-complex tachycardia* consistent with unstable polymorphic ventricular tachycardia (irregular form and rate) should be treated with high-energy unsynchronized dose used for ventricular fibrillation: 360 J monophasic waveform or biphasic device-specific defibrillation dose. |

(continued)

## Cardioversion
(Synchronized)

*(continued)*

- Some defibrillators cannot deliver synchronized cardioversion unless the patient is also connected to monitor leads; in other defibrillators, electrocardiogram leads are incorporated into the defibrillation pads. Lead select switch may need to be on *lead I, II, or III* and not on *paddles*.

- Press *charge* button, clear the patient, and press both *shock* buttons simultaneously. Be prepared to perform CPR or defibrillation.

---

## Transcutaneous pacing
Generally external pacemakers allow adjustment of heart rate and current outputs

### Indications
- Unstable bradycardia (<50/min) with signs and symptoms related to the bradycardia (hypotension, acutely altered mental status, signs of shock, ischemic chest discomfort, or acute heart failure) unresponsive to drug therapy.
- Be ready to pace in setting of acute myocardial infarction, as follows:
  - Markedly symptomatic sinus node dysfunction
  - Type II second-degree heart block
  - Third-degree heart block
  - New left, right, or alternating bundle branch block or bifascicular block
- Symptomatic bradycardia with ventricular escape rhythms.
- Not recommended for agonal rhythms or cardiac arrest.

### Precautions
- Conscious patients may require analgesia for discomfort.
- Avoid using carotid pulse to confirm mechanical capture. Electrical stimulation causes muscular jerking that may mimic carotid pulse.

### Technique
- Position pacing electrodes on chest per package instructions.
- Turn pacer on.
- Set demand rate to approximately 80/min.
- Set current (mA) output as follows for bradycardia: increase current from minimum setting until consistent capture is achieved (characterized by a widening QRS and a broad T wave after each pacer spike).

# Cardiac Arrest in Pregnancy In-Hospital ACLS Algorithm

**Continue BLS/ACLS**
- High-quality CPR
- Defibrillation when indicated
- Other ACLS interventions (eg, epinephrine)

↓

**Assemble maternal cardiac arrest team**

↓

**Consider etiology of arrest**

**Perform maternal interventions**
- Perform airway management
- Administer 100% O₂, avoid excess ventilation
- Place IV above diaphragm
- If receiving IV magnesium, stop and give calcium chloride or gluconate

**Perform obstetric interventions**
- Provide continuous lateral uterine displacement
- Detach fetal monitors
- Prepare for perimortem cesarean delivery

### Maternal Cardiac Arrest

- Team planning should be done in collaboration with the obstetric, neonatal, emergency, anesthesiology, intensive care, and cardiac arrest services.
- Priorities for pregnant women in cardiac arrest should include provision of high-quality CPR and relief of aortocaval compression with lateral uterine displacement.
- The goal of perimortem cesarean delivery is to improve maternal and fetal outcomes.
- Ideally, perform perimortem cesarean delivery in 5 minutes, depending on provider resources and skill sets.

### Advanced Airway

- In pregnancy, a difficult airway is common. Use the most experienced provider.
- Provide endotracheal intubation

**Continue BLS/ACLS**
- High-quality CPR
- Defibrillation when indicated
- Other ACLS interventions (eg, epinephrine)

**Perform perimortem cesarean delivery**
- If no ROSC, complete perimortem cesarean delivery ideally within 5 minutes after time of arrest

**Neonatal team to receive neonate**

- Perform waveform capnography or capnometry to confirm and monitor ET tube placement.
- Once advanced airway is in place, give 1 breath every 6 seconds (10 breaths/min) with continuous chest compressions.

**Potential Etiology of Maternal Cardiac Arrest**

A  Anesthetic complications

B  Bleeding

C  Cardiovascular

D  Drugs

E  Embolic

F  Fever

G  General nonobstetric causes of cardiac arrest (H's and T's)

H  Hypertension

Abbreviations: ACLS, advanced cardiovascular life support; BLS, basic life support; CPR, cardiopulmonary resuscitation; ET, endotracheal; IV, intravenous; ROSC, return of spontaneous circulation.

# Adult Suspected Stroke Algorithm

**Identify signs and symptoms of possible stroke**
Activate emergency response

↓

**Critical EMS assessments and actions**
- Assess ABCs; give oxygen if needed
- Perform physical exam
- Initiate stroke protocol
- Establish time of symptom onset (last known normal)
- Triage to most appropriate stroke center
- Check glucose; treat if indicated
- Perform validated prehospital stroke screen and stroke severity tool
- Provide prehospital notification; on arrival, transport to brain imaging suite

*Note: Refer to the expanded EMS stroke algorithm.*

↓

**ED or brain imaging suite***

**Immediate general and neurologic assessment by hospital or stroke team**
- Activate stroke team upon EMS notification
- Prepare for emergent CT scan or MRI of brain upon arrival
- Stroke team meets EMS on arrival
- Assess ABCs; give oxygen if needed
- Obtain IV access and perform laboratory assessments
- Check glucose; treat if indicated
- Review patient history, medications, and procedures
- Establish time of symptom onset or last known normal
- Perform physical exam and neurologic examination, including NIH Stroke Scale or Canadian Neurological Scale

*Best practice is to bypass the ED and go straight to the brain imaging suite.

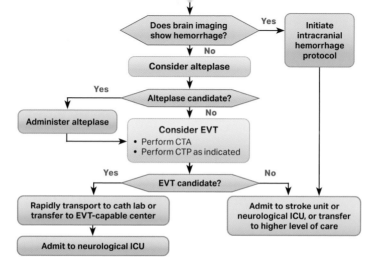

Abbreviations: ABCs, airway, breathing, circulation; CT, computed tomography; CTA, computed tomographic angiography; CTP, computed tomographic perfusion; ED, emergency department; EMS, emergency medical services; EVT, endovascular therapy; ICU, intensive care unit; IV, intravenous; MRI, magnetic resonance imaging, NIH, National Institutes of Health.

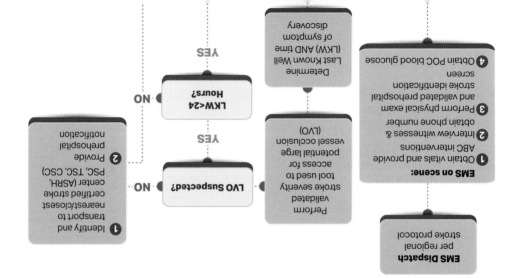

**EMS Dispatch**
per regional
stroke protocol

**EMS on scene:**
1. Obtain vitals and provide ABC interventions
2. Interview witnesses & obtain phone number
3. Perform physical exam and validated prehospital stroke identification screen
4. Obtain POC blood glucose

Perform validated stroke severity tool used to access for potential large vessel occlusion (LVO)

**LVO Suspected?**

NO

YES

**LKW<24 Hours?**

NO

YES

Determine Last Known Well (LKW) AND time of symptom discovery

1. Identify and transport to nearest closest certified stroke center (ASRH, PSC, TSC, CSC)
2. Provide prehospital notification

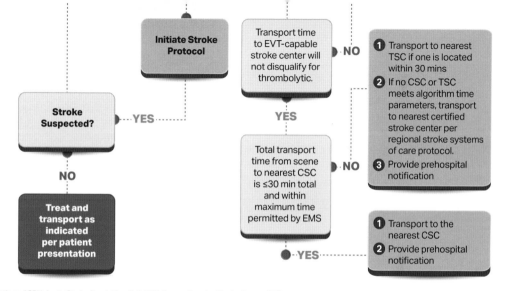

**Stroke Suspected?** — **YES** → **Initiate Stroke Protocol**

**Transport time to EVT-capable stroke center will not disqualify for thrombolytic.**

**NO** →
1. Transport to nearest TSC if one is located within 30 mins
2. If no CSC or TSC meets algorithm time parameters, transport to nearest certified stroke center per regional stroke systems of care protocol.
3. Provide prehospital notification

**YES** ↓

**Total transport time from scene to nearest CSC is ≤30 min total and within maximum time permitted by EMS**

**NO** →
1. Transport to nearest TSC if one is located within 30 mins
2. If no CSC or TSC meets algorithm time parameters, transport to nearest certified stroke center per regional stroke systems of care protocol.
3. Provide prehospital notification

**YES** →
1. Transport to the nearest CSC
2. Provide prehospital notification

**Stroke Suspected?** — **NO** ↓

**Treat and transport as indicated per patient presentation**

Abbreviations: ASRH, Acute Stroke Ready Hospital ; CSC, Comprehensive Stroke Center; EMS, emergency medical services; EVT, endovascular thrombectomy; LKW, last known well; LVO, large-vessel occlusion; POC, point of care; PSC, Primary Stroke Center; TSC, Thrombectomy-Capable Stroke Center.

## The 8 D's of Stroke Care

The 8 D's of stroke care highlight the major steps in diagnosis and treatment of stroke and key points at which delays can occur:

| | |
|---|---|
| **Detection** | Rapid recognition of stroke signs and symptoms |
| **Dispatch** | Early activation and dispatch of emergency medical services system by calling 9-1-1 |
| **Delivery** | Rapid emergency medical services stroke identification, management, triage, and prehospital notification |
| **Door** | Emergent emergency department/imaging suite triage and immediate assessment by the stroke team |
| **Data** | Rapid clinical evaluation, laboratory testing, and brain imaging |
| **Decision** | Establishing stroke diagnosis and determining optimal therapy selection |
| **Drug/device** | Administration of fibrinolytic and/or endovascular therapy if eligible |
| **Disposition** | Rapid admission to the stroke unit or critical care unit, or emergent interfacility transfer for endovascular therapy |

Modified from Demystifying recognition and management of stroke. *Currents in Emergency Cardiac Care.* 1996;7(4):8.

# Out-of-Hospital Assessment of the Patient With Acute Stroke

- Perform initial assessment
  - Assess and support airway, breathing, and circulation as needed
  - Determine level of consciousness
  - Measure vital signs frequently
- Obtain relevant history
  - Identify time of symptom onset or last seen normal
  - Determine recent illness (including history of seizures), injury, surgery, and list of medications
- Perform physical examination
  - Conduct general medical examination (including search for cardiovascular abnormalities)
  - Determine blood glucose level
  - Observe for signs of trauma
  - Conduct neurologic examination
    - Review Glasgow Coma Scale.
    - Perform a rapid prehospital stroke screen (eg, Cincinnati Prehospital Stroke Scale, Los Angeles Prehospital Stroke Screen).
    - Perform the stroke severity assessment for possible large vessel occlusion (LVO) (eg, Los Angeles Motor Scale, Rapid Arterial Occlusion Evaluation, Cincinnati Stroke Triage Assessment Tool, Field Assessment Stroke Triage for Emergency Destination).
- Determine the time of symptom onset or when the patient was at last known normal or at neurologic baseline. This represents time zero. If the patient wakes from sleep with symptoms of stroke, time zero is the last time the patient was seen to be normal.
- Once possible stroke is identified
  - Provide prearrival notification to receiving hospital of potential stroke patient.
  - Patients with a positive stroke screen or who are strongly suspected to have a stroke should be transported rapidly to the closest healthcare facilities that are able to administer intravenous (IV) alteplase.
  - Effective prehospital procedures to identify patients who are ineligible for IV thrombolysis and have a strong probability of LVO stroke should be developed to facilitate rapid transport of patients potentially eligible for thrombectomy to the closest healthcare facilities that are able to perform mechanical thrombectomy.
  - Obtain family contact information (preferably a cell phone); bring family member or transport witness if possible.

## The Cincinnati Prehospital Stroke Scale

**Facial Droop** (have the patient show teeth or smile):

- **Normal**—both sides of face move equally
- **Abnormal**—one side of face does not move as well as the other side

**Arm Drift** (patient closes eyes and extends both arms straight out, with palms up, for 10 seconds):

- **Normal**—both arms move the same or both arms do not move at all (other findings, such as pronator drift, may be helpful)
- **Abnormal**—one arm does not move or one arm drifts down compared with the other

**Abnormal Speech** (have the patient say, "You can't teach an old dog new tricks"):

- **Normal**—patient uses correct words with no slurring
- **Abnormal**—patient slurs words, uses the wrong words, or is unable to speak

*Interpretation:* If any 1 of these 3 signs is abnormal, the probability of a stroke is 72%.

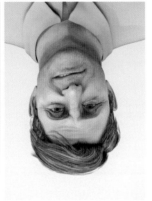

Stroke patient with facial droop
*(right side of face)*

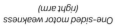

One-sided motor weakness
*(right arm)*

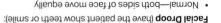

Modified from Kothari RU, Pancioli A, Liu T, Brott T, Broderick J. Cincinnati Prehospital Stroke Scale: reproducibility and

| Glasgow Coma Scale* | Score (maximum = 15) |
| --- | --- |
| **Eye opening** | |
| Spontaneous | 4 |
| In response to speech | 3 |
| In response to pain | 2 |
| None | 1 |
| **Best verbal response** | |
| Oriented conversation | 5 |
| Confused conversation | 4 |
| Inappropriate words | 3 |
| Incomprehensible sounds | 2 |
| None | 1 |
| **Best motor response** | |
| Obeys | 6 |
| Localizes | 5 |
| Withdraws | 4 |
| Abnormal flexion | 3 |
| Abnormal extension | 2 |
| None | 1 |

*Interpretation:*
**Score 14-15:** Mild dysfunction
**Score 11-13:** Moderate to severe dysfunction
**Score ≤10:** Severe dysfunction

### General management of the acute stroke patient

1. **Intravenous fluids:** Avoid $D_5W$ and excessive fluid loading. Correct hypovolemia with normal saline.

2. **Blood sugar:** Determine immediately. Bolus of 50% dextrose if hypoglycemic; administer insulin if serum glucose >185 mg/dL or administer glucose if serum glucose is <60 mg/dL (threshold varies; check institution/system protocol).

3. **Cardiac monitoring:** During first 24 hours.

4. **Oxygen:** Pulse oximetry. Supplement for oxyhemoglobin saturation ≤94%.

5. **Acetaminophen:** If febrile (temperature >38°C). Sources of hyperthermia (temperature >38°C) should be identified and treated, and antipyretic medications should be administered to lower temperature in hyperthermic patients with stroke.

6. **NPO:** Perform swallowing assessment.

Abbreviation: NPO, nil per os (nothing by mouth).

*Teasdale G, Jennett B. Assessment of coma and impaired consciousness: a practical scale. *Lancet.* 1974;2(7872):81-84.

# Use of IV Alteplase for Acute Ischemic Stroke: Inclusion and Exclusion Characteristics

**Inclusion and Exclusion Characteristics of Patients With Ischemic Stroke Who Could Be Treated With Alteplase Within 3 Hours After Symptom Onset and Extended Window for Select Patient From 3 to 4.5 Hours***

| Indications (COR 1) | |
|---|---|
| **Within 3 hours†** | IV alteplase (0.9 mg/kg, maximum dose 90 mg over 60 minutes with initial 10% of dose given as bolus over 1 minute) is recommended for selected patients who may be treated within 3 hours of ischemic stroke symptom onset or patient last known well or at baseline state. Physicians should review the criteria outlined in this table to determine patient eligibility.‡ (COR 1; LOE A) |
| **Within 3 hours—Age** | For otherwise medically eligible patients ≥18 years of age, IV alteplase administration within 3 hours is equally recommended for patients ≤80 and >80 years of age.‡ (COR 1; LOE A) |
| **Within 3 hours—Severe stroke** | For severe ischemic stroke, IV alteplase is indicated within 3 hours from symptom onset of ischemic stroke. Despite increased risk of hemorrhagic transformation, there is still proven clinical benefit for patients with severe stroke symptoms.‡ (COR 1; LOE A) |
| **Within 3 hours—Mild disabling stroke** | For otherwise eligible patients with mild but disabling stroke symptoms, IV alteplase is recommended for patients who can be treated within 3 hours of ischemic stroke symptom onset or patient last known well or at baseline state. (COR 1; LOE B-R)§ |
| **BP** | IV alteplase is recommended in those patients with BP < 185/110 mm Hg and in those patients whose BP can be lowered safely to this level with the physician assessing the stability of the BP before starting IV alteplase.‡ (COR 1; LOE B-NR)|| |
| **CT** | IV alteplase administration is recommended in the setting of early ischemic changes on NCCT of mild to moderate extent (other than frank hypodensity).‡ (COR 1; LOE A) |

| Additional recommendations for treatment with IV alteplase for patients with AIS (COR 2a) | And (COR 2b) |
|---|---|
| **Wake-up and unknown time of onset** | IV alteplase (0.9 mg/kg, maximum dose 90 mg over 60 minutes with initial 10% of dose given as bolus over 1 minute) administered within 4.5 hours of stroke symptom recognition can be beneficial in patients with AIS who awake with stroke symptoms or have unclear time of onset >4.5 hours from last known well or at baseline state and who have a DW-MRI lesion smaller than one third of the MCA territory and no visible signal change on FLAIR. (COR 2a; LOE B-R)§ |
| **Early improvement** | IV alteplase treatment is reasonable for patients who present with moderate to severe ischemic stroke and demonstrate early improvement but remain moderately impaired and potentially disabled in the judgment of the examiner.‡ (COR 2a; LOE A) |
| **Stroke mimics** | The risk of symptomatic intracranial hemorrhage in the stroke mimic population is quite low; thus, starting IV alteplase is probably recommended in preference over delaying treatment to pursue additional diagnostic studies.‡ (COR 2a; LOE B-NR)‖ |

| Contraindications (COR 3: No Benefit)* | And (COR 3: Harm) |
|---|---|
| **0 to 4.5-hour window—Mild nondisabling stroke** | For otherwise eligible patients with mild nondisabling stroke (NIHSS score 0–5), IV alteplase is not recommended for patients who could be treated within 3 and 4.5 hours of ischemic stroke symptom onset or patient last known well or at baseline state. (COR 3: No Benefit, LOE B-R)§ |

*(continued)*

# Use of IV Alteplase for Acute Ischemic Stroke: Inclusion and Exclusion Characteristics

| | Contraindications (COR 3: No Benefit)* And (COR 3: Harm) |
|---|---|
| CT | There remains insufficient evidence to identify a threshold of hypoattenuation severity or extent that affects treatment response to alteplase. However, administering IV alteplase to patients whose CT brain imaging exhibits extensive regions of clear hypoattenuation is not recommended. These patients have a poor prognosis despite IV alteplase, and severe hypoattenuation defined as obvious hypodensity represents irreversible injury.‡ (COR 3: No Benefit; LOE A)¶ |
| ICH | IV alteplase should not be administered to a patient whose CT reveals an acute intracranial hemorrhage.‡ (COR 3: Harm; LOE C-EO)¶ |
| Ischemic stroke within 3 months | Use of IV alteplase in patients presenting with AIS who have had a prior ischemic stroke within 3 months may be harmful.‡ (COR 3: Harm; LOE B-NR)¶ |
| Severe head trauma within 3 months | In AIS patients with recent severe head trauma (within 3 months), IV alteplase is contraindicated.‡ (COR 3: Harm; LOE C-EO)¶ |
| Acute head trauma | Given the possibility of bleeding complications from the underlying severe head trauma, IV alteplase should not be administered in posttraumatic infarction that occurs during the acute in-hospital phase.‡ (COR 3: Harm; LOE C-EO)¶ (Recommendation wording modified to match COR 3 stratifications.) |
| Intracranial/intraspinal surgery within 3 months | For patients with AIS and a history of intracranial/spinal surgery within the prior 3 months, IV alteplase is potentially harmful.‡ (COR 3: Harm; LOE C-EO)¶ |
| History of intracranial hemorrhage | IV alteplase administration in patients who have a history of intracranial hemorrhage is potentially harmful.‡ (COR 3: Harm; LOE C-EO)¶ |

(continued)

| Contraindications (COR 3: No Benefit)* | And (COR 3: Harm) |
|---|---|
| **Subarachnoid hemorrhage** | IV alteplase is contraindicated in patients presenting with symptoms and signs most consistent with an SAH.‡ (COR 3: Harm; LOE C-EO)‖¶ |
| **GI malignancy or GI bleed within 21 days** | Patients with a structural GI malignancy or recent bleeding event within 21 days of their stroke event should be considered high risk, and IV alteplase administration is potentially harmful.‡ (COR 3: Harm; LOE C-EO)‖¶ |
| **Coagulopathy** | The safety and efficacy of IV alteplase for acute stroke patients with platelets <100 000/mm³, INR >1.7, aPTT >40 seconds, or PT >15 seconds are unknown, and IV alteplase should not be administered.‡ (COR 3: Harm; LOE C-EO)‖¶ |
| | (In patients without history of thrombocytopenia, treatment with IV alteplase can be initiated before availability of platelet count but should be discontinued if platelet count is <100 000/mm³. In patients without recent use of OACs or heparin, treatment with IV alteplase can be initiated before availability of coagulation test results but should be discontinued if INR is >1.7 or PT is abnormally elevated by local laboratory standards.) (Recommendation wording modified to match COR 3 stratifications.) |
| **LMWH** | IV alteplase should not be administered to patients who have received a full treatment dose of LMWH within the previous 24 hours.‡ (COR 3: Harm; LOE B-NR)§‖ |
| | (Recommendation wording modified to match COR 3 stratifications.) |
| **Thrombin inhibitors or factor Xa inhibitors** | The use of IV alteplase in patients taking direct thrombin inhibitors or direct factor Xa inhibitors has not been firmly established but may be harmful.‡ (COR 3: Harm; LOE C-EO)‖¶ IV alteplase should not be administered to patients taking direct thrombin inhibitors or direct factor Xa inhibitors unless laboratory tests such as aPTT, INR, platelet count, ecarin clotting time, thrombin time, or appropriate direct factor Xa activity assays are normal or the patient has not received a dose of these agents for >48 hours (assuming normal renal metabolizing function). |
| | (Alteplase could be considered when appropriate laboratory tests such as aPTT, INR, ecarin clotting time, thrombin time, or direct factor Xa activity assays are normal or when the patient has not taken a dose of these ACs for >48 hours and renal function is normal.) (Recommendation wording modified to match COR 3 stratifications.) |
| **Concomitant abciximab** | Abciximab should not be administered concurrently with IV alteplase. (COR 3: Harm; LOE B-R)§ |

**Alteplase Considerations in the 3- to 4.5-Hour Time Window in Addition to Those in the 0- to 3-Hour Window\***

| Indications (COR 1) | |
|---|---|
| 3-4.5 hours† | IV alteplase (0.9 mg/kg, maximum dose 90 mg over 60 min with initial 10% of dose given as bolus over 1 min) is also recommended for selected patients who can be treated within 3 and 4.5 hours of ischemic stroke symptom onset or patient last known well. Physicians should review the criteria outlined in this table to determine patient eligibility.‡ (COR 1; LOE B-R)\|| |
| 3-4.5 hours–Age | IV alteplase treatment in the 3- to 4.5-hour time window is recommended for those patients ≤80 years of age, without a history of both diabetes mellitus and prior stroke, NIHSS score ≤25, not taking any OACs, and without imaging evidence of ischemic injury involving more than one third of the MCA territory.‡ (COR 1; LOE B-R)\|| |

| Additional recommendations for treatment with IV alteplase for patients with AIS (COR 2a) | And (COR 2b) |
|---|---|
| 3-4.5 hours–Age | For patients >80 years of age presenting in the 3- to 4.5-hour window, IV alteplase is safe and can be as effective as in younger patients.‡ (COR 2a; LOE B-NR)\|| |
| 3-4.5 hours—Diabetes mellitus and prior stroke | In AIS patients with prior stroke and diabetes mellitus presenting in the 3- to 4.5- hour window, IV alteplase may be as effective as treatment in the 0- to 3-hour window and may be a reasonable option.‡ (COR 2b; LOE B-NR)\|| |

*(continued)*

| Additional recommendations for treatment with IV alteplase for patients with AIS (COR 2a) | And (COR 2b) |
|---|---|
| 3-4.5 hours—Severe stroke | The benefit of IV alteplase between 3 and 4.5 hours from symptom onset for patients with very severe stroke symptoms (NIHSS score >25) is uncertain.‡ (COR 2b; LOE C-LD)‖ |
| 3 -4.5 hours—Mild disabling stroke | For otherwise eligible patients with mild disabling stroke, IV alteplase may be reasonable for patients who can be treated within 3 and 4.5 hours of ischemic stroke symptom onset or patient last known well or at baseline state. (COR 2b; LOE B-NR)§ |

Abbreviations: AC, anticoagulants; AIS, acute ischemic stroke; aPTT, activated partial thromboplastin time; BP, blood pressure; COR, Class of Recommendation; CT, computed tomography; DW-MRI, diffusion-weighted magnetic resonance imaging; FLAIR, fluid-attenuated inversion recovery; GI, gastrointestinal; ICH, intracerebral hemorrhage; INR, international normalized ratio; IV, intravenous; LMWH, low-molecular-weight heparin; LOE, Level of Evidence; MCA, middle cerebral artery; NCCT, noncontrast computed tomography; NIHSS, National Institutes of Health Stroke Scale; OAC, oral anticoagulant; PT, prothromboplastin time.

*The relative contraindications are abbreviated. Modified from Table 8 in Powers WJ, Rabinstein AA, Ackerson T, et al. Guidelines for the early management of patients with acute ischemic stroke: 2019 update to the 2018 guidelines for the early management of acute ischemic stroke: a guideline for healthcare professionals from the American Heart Association/American Stroke Association. *Stroke.* 2019;50(12):e344-e418. Please see Table 8 for a full listing of specific considerations.

†When uncertain, the time of onset time should be considered the time when the patient was last known to be normal or at baseline neurological condition.

‡Recommendation unchanged or reworded for clarity from 2015 IV Alteplase. See Table XCV in online Data Supplement 1 for original wording.

§See also the text of these guidelines for additional information on these recommendations.

‖LOE amended to conform with American College of Cardiology/AHA 2015 Recommendation Classification System.

¶COR amended to conform with American College of Cardiology/AHA 2015 Recommendation Classification System.

Clinicians should also be informed of the indications and contraindications from local regulatory agencies (for current information from the US Food and Drug Administration, refer to **http://www.accessdata.fda.gov/drugsatfda_docs/label/2015/103172s5203lbl.pdf**).

For a detailed discussion of this topic and evidence supporting these recommendations, refer to Demaerschalk BM, Kleindorfer DO, Adeoye OM, et al. Scientific rationale for the inclusion and exclusion criteria for intravenous alteplase in acute ischemic stroke: a statement for healthcare professionals from the American Heart Association/American Stroke Association. *Stroke.* 2016;47:581-641.

## Options to Treat Arterial Hypertension in Patients with Acute Ischemic Stroke Who Are Candidates for Emergency Reperfusion Therapy*

| COR 2b | LOE C-EO |
|---|---|
| Patient otherwise eligible for emergency reperfusion therapy except that BP is >185/110 mm Hg:<br>• Labetalol 10-20 mg IV over 1-2 minutes, may repeat 1 time; or<br>• Nicardipine 5 mg/h IV, titrate up by 2.5 mg/h every 5-15 minutes, maximum 15 mg/h; when desired BP reached, adjust to maintain proper BP limits; or<br>• Clevidipine 1-2 mg/h IV, titrate by doubling the dose every 2-5 minutes until desired BP reached; maximum 21 mg/h<br>• Other agents (eg, hydralazine, enalaprilat) may also be considered<br>• If BP is not maintained ≤185/110 mm Hg, do not administer alteplase | |
| Management of BP during and after alteplase or other emergency reperfusion therapy to maintain BP ≤180/105 mm Hg:<br>• Monitor BP every 15 minutes for 2 hours from the start of alteplase therapy, then every 30 minutes for 6 hours, and then every hour for 16 hours | |
| If systolic BP >180-230 mm Hg or diastolic BP > 105-120 mm Hg:<br>• Labetalol 10 mg IV followed by continuous IV infusion 2-8 mg/min; or<br>• Nicardipine 5 mg/h IV, titrate up to desired effect by 2.5 mg/h every 5-15 minutes, maximum 15 mg/h; or<br>• Clevidipine 1-2 mg/h IV, titrate by doubling the dose every 2-5 minutes until desired BP reached; maximum 21 mg/h<br>• If BP not controlled or diastolic BP >140 mm Hg, consider IV sodium nitroprusside | |

Abbreviations: BP, blood pressure; COR, Class of Recommendation; IV, intravenous; LOE, Level of Evidence.

*Different treatment options may be appropriate in patients who have comorbid conditions that may benefit from rapid reductions in BP, such as acute coronary heart failure, aortic dissection, or preeclampsia/eclampsia.

Reprinted from Powers WJ, Rabinstein AA, Ackerson T, et al. Guidelines for the early management of patients with acute ischemic stroke: 2019 update to the 2018 guidelines for the early management of acute ischemic stroke: a guideline for healthcare professionals from the American Heart Association/American Stroke Association. *Stroke*. 2019;50(12):e344-e418. Data derived from Jauch EC, Saver JL, Adams HP Jr, et al; Guidelines for the early management of patients with acute ischemic stroke: a guideline for healthcare professionals from the American Heart Association/American Stroke Association. *Stroke*. 2013;44(3):870-947.

# Acute Coronary Syndromes Algorithm

**Symptoms suggestive of ischemia or infarction**

**EMS assessment and care and hospital preparation**
- Assess ABCs. Be prepared to provide CPR and defibrillation
- Administer aspirin and consider oxygen, nitroglycerin, and morphine if needed
- Obtain 12-lead ECG; if ST elevation:
  – Notify receiving hospital with transmission or interpretation; note time of onset and first medical contact
- Provide prehospital notification; on arrival, transport to ED/cath lab per protocol
- Notified hospital should mobilize resources to respond to STEMI
- If considering prehospital fibrinolysis, use fibrinolytic checklist

**Concurrent ED/cath lab assessment (<10 minutes)**
- Activate STEMI team upon EMS notification
- Assess ABCs; give oxygen if needed
- Establish IV access
- Perform brief, targeted history, physical exam
- Review/complete fibrinolytic checklist; check contraindications
- Obtain initial cardiac marker levels, complete blood counts, and coagulation studies
- Obtain portable chest x-ray (<30 minutes); do not delay transport to the cath lab

**Immediate ED/cath lab general treatment**
- If O₂ sat <90%, start oxygen at 4 L/min, titrate
- **Aspirin** 162 to 325 mg (if not given by EMS)
- **Nitroglycerin** sublingual or translingual
- **Morphine** IV if discomfort not relieved by nitroglycerin
- Consider administration of **P2Y₁₂ inhibitors**

**ECG interpretation**

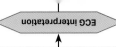

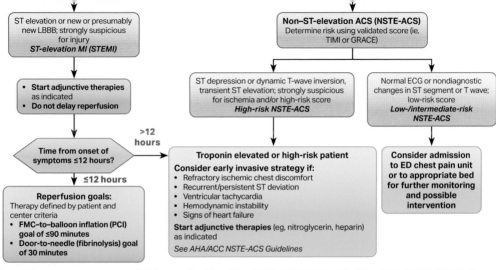

ST elevation or new or presumably new LBBB; strongly suspicious for injury
***ST-elevation MI (STEMI)***

- Start adjunctive therapies as indicated
- **Do not delay reperfusion**

**Time from onset of symptoms ≤12 hours?**

>12 hours

≤12 hours

**Reperfusion goals:**
Therapy defined by patient and center criteria
- **FMC–to–balloon inflation (PCI) goal of ≤90 minutes**
- **Door-to-needle (fibrinolysis) goal of 30 minutes**

**Non–ST-elevation ACS (NSTE-ACS)**
Determine risk using validated score (ie, TIMI or GRACE)

ST depression or dynamic T-wave inversion, transient ST elevation; strongly suspicious for ischemia and/or high-risk score
***High-risk NSTE-ACS***

Normal ECG or nondiagnostic changes in ST segment or T wave; low-risk score
***Low-/intermediate-risk NSTE-ACS***

**Troponin elevated or high-risk patient**
**Consider early invasive strategy if:**
- Refractory ischemic chest discomfort
- Recurrent/persistent ST deviation
- Ventricular tachycardia
- Hemodynamic instability
- Signs of heart failure

**Start adjunctive therapies** (eg, nitroglycerin, heparin) as indicated
*See AHA/ACC NSTE-ACS Guidelines*

**Consider admission to ED chest pain unit or to appropriate bed for further monitoring and possible intervention**

Abbreviations: ACS, acute coronary syndromes; AHA, American Heart Association; ACC, American College of Cardiology; ECG, electrocardiogram; ED, emergency department; EMS, emergency medical services; FMC, first medical contact; GRACE, Global Registry of Acute Cardiac Events; IV, intravenous; LBBB, left bundle branch block; NSTE-ACS, non–ST-elevation acute coronary syndromes; PCI, percutaneous coronary intervention; STEMI, ST-segment elevation myocardial infarction; TIMI, thrombolysis in myocardial infarction.

## Likelihood That Signs and Symptoms Represent an Acute Coronary Syndromes Secondary to Coronary Artery Disease

| Feature | High Likelihood<br>Any of the following: | Intermediate Likelihood<br>Absence of high-likelihood features and presence of any of the following: | Low Likelihood<br>Absence of high- or intermediate-likelihood features but may have the following: |
|---|---|---|---|
| History | Chest or left arm pain or discomfort as chief symptom reproducing prior documented angina<br>Known history of CAD, including MI | Chest or left arm pain or discomfort as chief symptom<br>Age > 70 years<br>Male sex<br>Diabetes mellitus | Probable ischemic symptoms in absence of any intermediate-likelihood characteristics<br>Recent cocaine use |
| Examination | Transient MR murmur, hypotension, diaphoresis, pulmonary edema, or rales | Extracardiac vascular disease | Chest discomfort reproduced by palpation |

(continued)

| Feature | **High Likelihood**<br>Any of the following: | **Intermediate Likelihood**<br>Absence of high-likelihood features and presence of any of the following: | **Low Likelihood**<br>Absence of high- or intermediate-likelihood features but may have the following: |
|---|---|---|---|
| **ECG** | New or presumably new transient ST-segment deviation (≥1 mm) or T-wave inversion in multiple precordial leads | Fixed Q waves<br>ST depression 0.5-1 mm or T-wave inversion >1 mm | T-wave flattening or inversion <1 mm in leads with dominant R waves<br>Normal ECG |
| **Cardiac markers** | Elevated cardiac TnI, TnT, CK-MB, hs-TnI, or hs-TnT | Normal | Normal |

Abbreviations: CAD, coronary artery disease; CK-MB, MB fraction of creatine kinase; ECG, electrocardiogram; hs, high-sensitivity; MI, myocardial infarction; MR, mitral regurgitation; TnI, troponin I; TnT, troponin T.

Anderson JL, Adams CD, Antman EM, et al. 2011 ACCF/AHA Focused Update Incorporated Into the 2007 ACC/AHA guidelines for the management of patients with unstable angina/non–ST-elevation myocardial infarction: a report of the American College of Cardiology Foundation/American Heart Association Task Force on Practice Guidelines. *Circulation.* 2011;123(18):e426-e579. Modified from Braunwald E, Mark DB, Jones RH, et al. *Unstable Angina: Diagnosis and Management.* Clinical Practice Guideline No. 10. Agency for Health Care Policy and Research and the National Heart, Lung, and Blood Institute, Public Health Service, US Department of Health and Human Services; 1994. AHCPR publication 94-0602.

## Triage and Assessment of Cardiac Risk in the Emergency Department/Cath Lab

### Stratifying Patients With Possible or Probable ACS in the ED/Cath Lab

- **Protocols must be in place to stratify** chest pain patients by risk of ACS. The 12-lead ECG is central to ED triage of **patients with ACS.** Stratify patients into one of the following subgroups (also see below):

  1. **ST-segment elevation or new left bundle branch block (LBBB): High specificity for evolving STEMI;** assess reperfusion eligibility.

  2. **Non–ST-elevation ACS (NSTE-ACS):**

     - **ST-segment depression:** Consistent with/strongly suggestive of ischemia; defines a high-risk subset of patients with NSTE-ACS. Especially important if there are new or dynamic ECG changes. Clinical correlation is necessary to interpret completely.

     - **Nondiagnostic or normal ECG:** Further assessment usually needed; evaluation protocols should include repeat ECG or continuous ST-segment monitoring and serial cardiac markers. Myocardial imaging or 2D echocardiogram may be useful during medical observation in selected patients. Noninvasive testing (ie, stress test/cardiac imaging) may be considered if ECG and serial markers remain normal.

- **Clinicians should carefully consider the diagnosis of ACS even in the absence of typical chest discomfort.** **Consider ACS in patients with**

  - Anginal equivalent symptoms, such as dyspnea (LV dysfunction), palpitations, presyncope, and syncope (ischemic ventricular arrhythmias)
  - Atypical left precordial pain or complaint of indigestion or dyspepsia
  - Atypical pain in the elderly, women, and persons with diabetes

- **Continually consider other causes of chest pain:** aortic dissection, pericarditis/myocarditis, pulmonary embolus

- **Fibrinolytic therapy:** When used for STEMI, administer within 30 minutes after hospital arrival

**Percutaneous coronary intervention (PCI).** Identify reperfusion candidates promptly and achieve balloon inflation as soon as possible with primary PCI; ideal first medical contact–to–balloon inflation time system goal of 90 minutes or less if transported directly to a PCI-capable hospital and 120 minutes or less if initially seen at a non–PCI-capable hospital

## Emergency Department Triage Recommendations

- **Symptoms and signs indicating need for immediate assessment and ECG within 10 minutes after presentation**
  - Chest or epigastric discomfort, nontraumatic in origin with components typical for ischemia or MI
  - Central substernal compression or crushing pain; pressure, tightness, heaviness, cramping, burning, aching sensation; unexplained indigestion, belching, epigastric pain; radiating pain in neck, jaws, shoulders, back, or one or both arms
  - Associated dyspnea, nausea or vomiting, diaphoresis
  - Palpitations, irregular pulse, or suspected arrhythmia
- **For all patients with ischemic-type chest pain**
  - Provide supplemental oxygen (until stable, for saturation less than 90%), IV access, and continuous ECG monitoring
  - Prompt interpretation of 12-lead ECG by physician responsible for ACS triage
- **For all patients with STEMI**
  - Initiate protocol for reperfusion therapy (fibrinolytics or PCI)
  - If fibrinolysis is planned, rule out contraindications and assess risk-benefit ratio
  - Primary PCI is the recommended method of reperfusion, including for patients considered ineligible for fibrinolytics
  - PCI (or coronary artery bypass grafting [CABG] if indicated) is the preferred reperfusion treatment for patients presenting in cardiogenic shock
- **For all patients with moderate- to high-risk NSTE-ACS and STEMI**
  - Prompt aspirin unless given in past 24 hours
  - Give P2Y$_{12}$ inhibitor such as clopidogrel, prasugrel, or ticagrelor
  - Start anticoagulation. See AHA/ACC STEMI and NSTE-ACS Guidelines.
- **Consider IV nitroglycerin for initial 24 to 48 hours only in patients with AMI and CHF, large anterior infarction, recurrent or persistent ischemia, or hypertension**

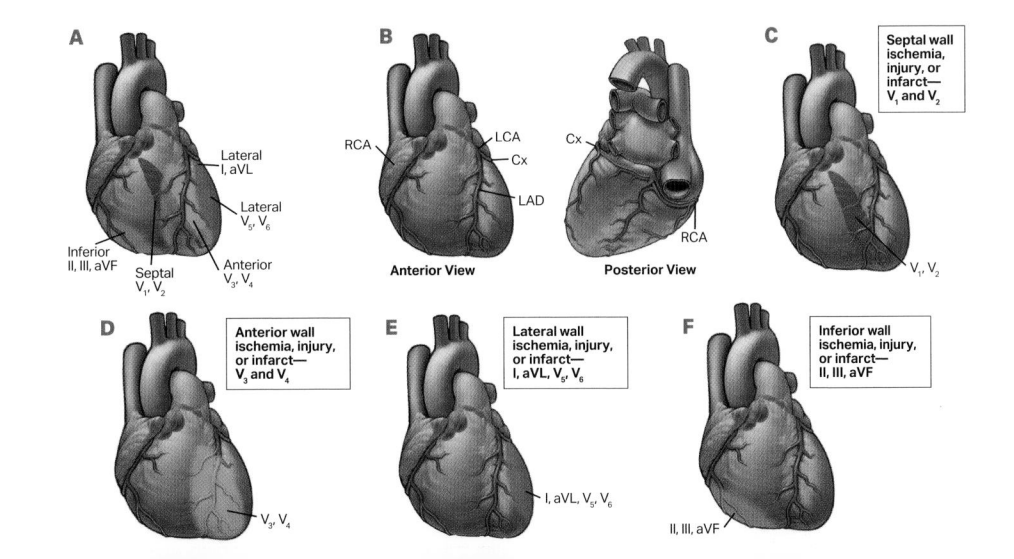

**A**

Lateral
I, aVL

Lateral
V₅, V₆

Inferior
II, III, aVF

Septal
V₁, V₂

Anterior
V₃, V₄

**B**

RCA

LCA
Cx
LAD

**Anterior View**

Cx

RCA

**Posterior View**

**C**

Septal wall
ischemia,
injury, or
infarct—
V₁ and V₂

V₁, V₂

**D**

Anterior wall
ischemia,
injury, or
infarct—
V₃ and V₄

V₃, V₄

**E**

Lateral wall
ischemia,
injury, or
infarct—
I, aVL, V₅, V₆

I, aVL, V₅, V₆

**F**

Inferior wall
ischemia,
injury, or
infarct—
II, III, aVF

II, III, aVF

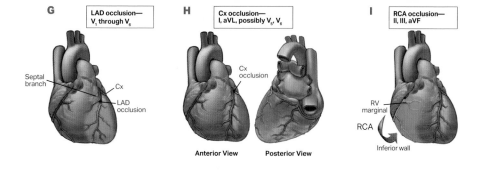

| G | LAD occlusion—V$_1$ through V$_6$ | H | Cx occlusion—I, aVL, possibly V$_5$, V$_6$ | I | RCA occlusion—II, III, aVF |

| I lateral | aVR | V$_1$ septal | V$_4$ anterior |
|-----------|-----|--------------|----------------|
| II inferior | aVL lateral | V$_2$ septal | V$_5$ lateral |
| III inferior | aVF inferior | V$_3$ anterior | V$_6$ lateral |

Localizing ischemia, injury, or infarct using the 12-lead ECG: relationship to coronary artery anatomy.

## How to Measure ST-Segment Deviation

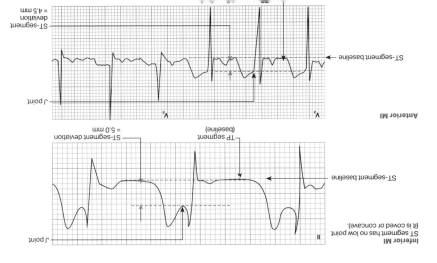

## ECG Lead Changes Due to Injury or Infarct With Coronary Artery, Anatomical Area of Damage, and Associated Complications

| Leads With ECG Changes | Injury/Infarct-Related Artery | Area of Damage | Associated Complications |
|---|---|---|---|
| $V_1$-$V_2$ | LCA: LAD-septal branch | Septum, His bundle, bundle branches | Infranodal block and BBBs |
| $V_3$-$V_4$ | LCA: LAD-diagonal branch | Anterior wall LV | LV dysfunction, CHF, BBBs, complete heart block, PVCs |
| $V_5$-$V_6$ plus I and aVL | LCA: circumflex branch | High lateral wall LV | LV dysfunction, AV nodal block in some |
| II, III, aVF | RCA: posterior descending branch | Inferior wall LV, posterior wall LV | Hypotension, sensitivity to nitroglycerin and morphine sulfate |
| $V_4$R (II, III, aVF) | RCA: proximal branches | RV, inferior wall LV, posterior wall LV | Hypotension, supranodal and AV-nodal blocks, atrial fibrillation/flutter, PACs, adverse medical reactions |
| $V_1$ through $V_4$ (marked depression) | Either LCA-circumflex or RCA-posterior descending branch | Posterior wall LV | LV dysfunction |

Abbreviations: AV, atrioventricular; BBB, bundle branch block; CHF, congestive heart failure; ECG, electrocardiographic; LAD, left anterior descending artery; LCA, left coronary artery; LV, left ventricle (left ventricular); PAC, premature atrial complex; PVC, premature ventricular complex; RCA, right coronary artery; RV, right ventricle.

# Acute Coronary Syndromes: ST-Segment Elevation Therapies: Evaluation for Reperfusion

## ST-Segment Elevation or New or Presumably New LBBB: Evaluation for Reperfusion

### Step 1: Assess time and risk

- Time since onset of symptoms
- Early risk assessment (TIMI or GRACE risk score)
- Risk of fibrinolysis
- Assess bleeding risk
- Time required to transport to skilled PCI catheterization suite (first medical contact/door-to-balloon time)

### Step 2: Select reperfusion (invasive or fibrinolysis) strategy

**Note: if presentation 3 hours or less from symptom onset and no delay for PCI, then PCI is the preferred strategy.**

**Fibrinolysis is generally preferred if**

- Early presentation (3 hours from symptom onset)
- Invasive strategy is not an option (eg, lack of access to skilled PCI facility or difficult vascular access) or would be delayed
- First medical contact–to–balloon inflation time is greater than 90 minutes

**An invasive strategy is generally preferred if**

- No contraindications to fibrinolysis
- Late presentation (symptom onset more than 3 hours ago)

- First medical contact–to–balloon inflation time 90 min or less
- Contraindications to fibrinolysis, including increased risk of bleeding and ICH
- High risk from STEMI (eg, presenting in shock or congestive heart failure)
- Diagnosis of STEMI is in doubt

## Evaluate for Primary PCI

**Can restore vessel patency and normal flow with more than 90% success in experienced high-volume centers with experienced providers**

**Primary PCI is most effective for the following:**

- In cardiogenic shock patients (younger than 75 years old) if performed 18 hours or less from onset of shock and 36 hours or less from onset of ST-elevation infarction. However, up to 40% of shock patients require CABG for optimal management.
- In selected patients older than 75 years with STEMI and cardiogenic shock.
- In patients with indications for reperfusion but with a contraindication to fibrinolytic therapy.

**Best results achieved at PCI centers with these characteristics:**

- Centers with high volume (more than 200 PCI procedures per year; at least 36 are primary PCI)
- Experienced operator (more than 75 PCI procedures per year) with technical skill
- Balloon dilation less than 90 minutes from initial medical contact
- Achievement of normal flow rate (TIMI grade 3) in more than 90% of cases without emergency CABG, stroke, or death
  - At least 50% resolution of maximal ST-segment elevation (microvascular reperfusion)

## Update: Universal Definition of Acute Myocardial Infarction (Type 1)

Detection of a rise and/or fall of cTn values with at least 1 value above the 99th percentile URL and with at least 1 of the following:

- Symptoms of acute myocardial ischemia
- New ischemic ECG changes
- Development of pathological Q waves
- Imaging evidence of new loss of viable myocardium or new regional wall motion abnormality in a pattern consistent with an ischemic etiology
- Identification of a coronary thrombus by angiography including intracoronary imaging or by autopsy

### Cardiac Troponins

- Troponin I and troponin T are cardiac-specific structural proteins not normally detected in serum. Patients with increased troponin levels have increased thrombus burden and microvascular embolization.
- Preferred biomarker for diagnosis of MI. Increased sensitivity compared with CK-MB. Elevation above 99th percentile of mean population value is diagnostic.
- Detect minimal myocardial damage in patients with NSTE-ACS.
  - 30% of patients without ST-segment elevation who would otherwise be diagnosed with UA have small amounts of myocardial damage when troponin assays are used (eg, CK-MB negative).
  - These patients are at increased risk for major adverse cardiac events and may benefit from therapies such as GP IIb/IIIa inhibitors compared with patients who lack elevations in these cardiac-specific markers

- Useful in risk stratification because patients with elevated serum troponin concentrations are at increased risk for subsequent nonfatal MI and sudden cardiac death.
- Can also be used to detect reinfarction.
  - Remain elevated for 7 to 14 days after infarct.

## CK-MB

- Present in skeletal muscle and serum, less specific than troponin.
- Marker for reinfarction and noninvasive assessment of reperfusion.

## TIMI Risk Score for Patients With Unstable Angina and Non–ST-Segment Elevation MI: Predictor Variables

| Predictor Variable | Point Value of Variable | Definition |
|---|---|---|
| Age ≥65 years | 1 | |
| ≥3 risk factors for CAD | 1 | **Risk factors:**<br>• Family history of CAD<br>• Hypertension<br>• Hypercholesterolemia<br>• Diabetes<br>• Current smoker |
| Aspirin use in last 7 days | 1 | |
| Recent, severe symptoms of angina | 1 | ≥2 anginal events in last 24 hours |
| Elevated cardiac markers | 1 | CK-MB or cardiac-specific troponin level |

*(continued)*

| ST deviation ≥0.5 mm | 1 | ST depression ≥0.5 mm is significant; transient ST elevation ≥0.5 mm for <20 minutes is treated as ST-segment depression and is high risk; ST elevation >1 mm for more than 20 minutes places these patients in the STEMI treatment category. |
| **Prior coronary artery stenosis ≥50%** | 1 | Risk predictor remains valid even if this information is unknown. |

| Calculated TIMI Risk Score | Risk of ≥1 Primary End Point* in ≤14 Days | Risk Status |
|---|---|---|
| 0 or 1 | 5% | Low |
| 2 | 8% | Low |
| 3 | 13% | Intermediate |
| 4 | 20% | Intermediate |
| 5 | 26% | High |

Abbreviations: CAD, coronary artery disease; STEMI, ST-segment elevation myocardial infarction.

*Primary end points: death, new or recurrent MI, or need for urgent revascularization.
Antman EM, Cohen M, Bernink PJ, et al. The TIMI risk score for unstable angina/non-ST elevation MI: a method for prognostication and therapeutic decision making. *JAMA*. 2000;284(7):835-842.

# Acute Coronary Syndromes: GRACE Risk Calculator for In-Hospital Mortality

## Global Registry of Acute Coronary Events (GRACE) Risk Model Nomogram

1. Find points for each predictive factor:

| Killip Class | Points | SBP (mm Hg) | Points | Heart Rate (/min) | Points | Age (y) | Points | Creatinine Level (mg/dL) | Points |
|---|---|---|---|---|---|---|---|---|---|
| I | 0 | ≤80 | 58 | ≤50 | 0 | ≤30 | 0 | 0-0.39 | 1 |
| II | 20 | 80-99 | 53 | 50-69 | 3 | 30-39 | 8 | 0.40-0.79 | 4 |
| III | 39 | 100-119 | 43 | 70-89 | 6 | 40-49 | 25 | 0.80-1.19 | 7 |
| IV | 59 | 120-139 | 34 | 90-109 | 15 | 50-59 | 41 | 1.20-1.59 | 10 |
|  |  | 140-159 | 24 | 110-149 | 24 | 60-69 | 58 | 1.60-1.99 | 13 |
|  |  | 160-199 | 10 | 150-199 | 38 | 70-79 | 75 | 2.00-3.99 | 21 |
|  |  | ≥200 | 0 | ≥200 | 46 | 80-89 | 91 | <4.0 | 28 |
|  |  |  |  |  |  | ≥90 | 100 |  |  |

| Other Risk Factors | Points |
|---|---|
| Cardiac arrest at admission | 39 |
| ST-segment deviation | 28 |
| Elevated cardiac enzyme levels | 14 |

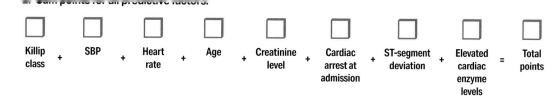

Sum points for all predictive factors:

Killip class + SBP + Heart rate + Age + Creatinine level + Cardiac arrest at admission + ST-segment deviation + Elevated cardiac enzyme levels = Total points

### 3. Look up risk corresponding to total points:

| Total points | ≤60 | 70 | 80 | 90 | 100 | 110 | 120 | 130 | 140 | 150 | 160 | 170 | 180 | 190 | 200 | 210 | 220 | 230 | 240 | ≥250 |
|---|---|---|---|---|---|---|---|---|---|---|---|---|---|---|---|---|---|---|---|---|
| Probability of in-hospital death (%) | ≤0.2 | 0.3 | 0.4 | 0.6 | 0.8 | 1.1 | 1.6 | 2.1 | 2.9 | 3.9 | 5.4 | 7.3 | 9.8 | 13 | 18 | 23 | 29 | 36 | 44 | ≥52 |

## P2Y$_{12}$ Inhibitors (also called *ADP Receptor Antagonists*)

Either clopidogrel or ticagrelor in addition to aspirin should be administered for up to 12 months to all patients with NSTE-ACS without contraindications who are treated with either an early invasive or ischemia-guided strategy.

A loading dose of a P2Y$_{12}$ inhibitor (any of the 3 below) should be given as early as possible or at the time of primary PCI to patients with STEMI or NSTE-ACS.

In patients receiving a stent during PCI for STEMI or NSTE-ACS, P2Y$_{12}$ inhibitor therapy should be given for at least 12 months.

### Clopidogrel

- Aspirin and clopidogrel (300 mg loading dose for patients 75 years of age or younger, 75 mg for patients older than 75 years of age) should be administered to patients with STEMI who receive fibrinolytic therapy.
- Aspirin should be continued indefinitely and clopidogrel (75 mg daily) should be continued for at least 14 days and up to 1 year in patients with STEMI who receive fibrinolytic therapy.
- For other indications, a loading dose of 300 to 600 mg is recommended, followed by 75 mg daily. A 600-mg loading dose results in a greater, more rapid, and more reliable platelet inhibition compared with a 300-mg loading dose.
- Clopidogrel is also recommended in patients with NSTE-ACS who are unable to take aspirin because of hypersensitivity or major gastrointestinal intolerance.
- When possible, discontinue clopidogrel at least 5 days before surgery.

- The recommended loading dose is 180 mg, followed by a maintenance dose of 90 mg twice daily.
- Compared with clopidogrel, ticagrelor has a more rapid and consistent onset of action and, because it is reversible, it has a faster recovery of platelet function. It is reasonable to choose ticagrelor over clopidogrel for $P2Y_{12}$ inhibition treatment in patients with NSTE-ACS treated with an early invasive strategy and/or coronary stenting.
- Although ticagrelor has not been studied in the absence of aspirin, its use in aspirin-intolerant patients is a reasonable alternative.
- When possible, discontinue ticagrelor at least 5 days before surgery.

## Prasugrel

- The recommended loading dose is 60 mg, followed by a maintenance dose of 10 mg daily.
- Prasugrel produces more rapid and consistent platelet inhibition than clopidogrel.
- A loading dose of prasugrel is reasonable once the coronary anatomy is known in STEMI patients who did not receive a previous loading dose of clopidogrel at the time of administration of a fibrinolytic agent, but prasugrel should not be given sooner than 24 hours after administration of a fibrin-specific agent or 48 hours after administration of a non–fibrin-specific agent.
- It is reasonable to choose prasugrel over clopidogrel for treatment in patients with NSTE-ACS who undergo PCI who are not at high risk of bleeding complications.
- Prasugrel is not recommended for "up-front" therapy in patients with NSTE-ACS.
- Prasugrel should not be administered to patients with a prior history of stroke or transient ischemic attack.
- When possible, discontinue prasugrel at least 7 days before surgery.

## Anticoagulants

- **STEMI–Fibrinolytic Adjunct:** Anticoagulant therapy for a minimum of 48 hours and preferably the duration of hospitalization, up to 8 days. Regimens other than unfractionated heparin (UFH) are recommended if anticoagulant therapy is given for more than 48 hours. Recommended regimens include

  – UFH: Initial bolus 60 units/kg (maximum 4000 units) followed by intravenous infusion of 12 units/kg per hour (maximum 1000 units per hour) initially adjusted to maintain the aPTT at 1.5 to 2× control (approximately 50 to 70 seconds). (duration of treatment 48 hours or until angiography).

  – Enoxaparin (if serum creatinine less than 2.5 mg/dL in men and 2 mg/dL in women): If age less than 75 years, an initial bolus of 30 mg IV is followed 15 minutes later by subcutaneous injections 1 mg/kg every 12 hours (maximum 100 mg for first 2 doses only). If age 75 years or older, the initial bolus is eliminated, and subcutaneous dose is reduced to 0.75 mg/kg every 12 hours (maximum 75 mg for first 2 doses only). Regardless of age, if creatinine clearance during course of treatment is estimated to be less than 30 mL/min (using Cockroft-Gault formula), the subcutaneous regimen is 1 mg/kg every 24 hours.

  – Patients initially treated with enoxaparin should not be switched to UFH and vice versa because of increased risk of bleeding.

  – Fondaparinux (provided serum creatinine less than 3 mg/dL and creatinine clearance 30 mL/min or greater): Initial dose 2.5 mg IV; subsequent subcutaneous injections 2.5 mg every 24 hours. Maintenance dosing should be continued for duration of hospitalization, up to 8 days.

- **NSTE-ACS:** For patients at high to intermediate risk, anticoagulant therapy should be added to antiplatelet therapy, initial invasive strategy.

- UFH: Use same as above.
- Enoxaparin: If creatinine clearance 30 mL/min or greater, give 1 mg/kg subcutaneously every 12 hours. If creatinine clearance less than 30 mL/min, give 1 mg/kg once every 24 hours. Patients initially treated with enoxaparin should not be switched to UFH and vice versa because of increased risk of bleeding.
- Fondaparinux: 2.5 mg subcutaneously every 24 hours. Contraindicated if creatinine clearance less than 30 mL/min.
- Bivalirudin: 0.1 mg/kg bolus; maintenance 0.25 mg/kg per hour infusion.

## Immediate General Treatment

- Oxygen
- Aspirin
- Nitroglycerin
- Morphine (if unresponsive to nitrates)

### Oxygen

If oxygen saturation less than 90% or evidence of respiratory distress: 4 L/min per nasal cannula; titrate to maintain $SaO_2$ 90% or greater.

- **Uncomplicated MI:** Reasonable to use until stabilization. May not be helpful beyond 6 hours.
- **Complicated MI** (for overt pulmonary congestion): Administer supplemental $O_2$ at 4 L/min by nasal cannula; titrate as needed.

### Aspirin

In either out-of-hospital or emergency department (ED)/cath lab setting, give aspirin to all patients with acute coronary syndromes (ACS) unless a true aspirin allergy exists (then consider clopidogrel).

#### Cautions and Contraindications

- Active peptic ulcer disease (use rectal suppositories).
- History of true aspirin allergy.
- Bleeding disorders, severe hepatic disease.

#### Recommended Dosing

- Give 162 to 325 mg non–enteric-coated orally, crushed or chewed (may use rectal suppository if cannot give by mouth).

## Nitroglycerin

Indicated for patients with ischemic-type chest pain.

### Cautions and Contraindications

- The use of nitrates in patients with hypotension (systolic blood pressure less than 90 mm Hg or 30 mm Hg or more below baseline), extreme bradycardia (less than 50/min), or tachycardia (greater than100/min) in the absence of heart failure is contraindicated.
- Administer nitrates with extreme caution, if at all, to patients with inferior wall MI and suspected right ventricular involvement, because these patients require adequate right ventricle (RV) preload. (Obtain right-sided electrocardiogram [ECG] leads to assist in diagnosing RV infarct.)
- Contraindicated in patients who have recently received a phosphodiesterase inhibitor (usually given for erectile dysfunction), especially within 24 hours after sildenafil or vardenafil, or within 48 hours after tadalafil.

### Recommended Dosing

- **SL:** 0.3 to 0.4 mg, repeat × 2 at 3- to 5-minute intervals, *or*
- **Spray:** 1 or 2 sprays, may repeat × 2 at 3- to 5-minute intervals, *or*
- **IV:** 12.5 to 25 mcg bolus (if no SL or spray given); then 10 mcg/min infusion, titrated (increased at a rate of 10 mcg/min every 3 to 5 minutes until symptom response or target arterial pressure is achieved). Ceiling dose of 200 mcg/min commonly used.

## Morphine

Indicated for patients with ischemic pain not relieved by nitroglycerin.

### Cautions and Contraindications

- Do not use in patients with hypotension.
- Use cautiously in patients with suspected hypovolemia, bradycardia, or known hypersensitivity.

### Recommended Dosing: STEMI

Give 2 to 4 mg IV; may give additional doses of 2 to 8 mg IV at 5- to 15-minute intervals.

### Recommended Dosing: Non-ST-Segment Elevation Acute Coronary Syndrome (NSTE-ACS)

Give 1 to 5 mg IV only if symptoms not relieved by nitrates, provided additional therapy is used to manage underlying ischemia.

Contraindications for fibrinolytic use in STEMI consistent with the 2013 ACCF/AHA Guideline for the Management of ST-Elevation Myocardial Infarction*

## Absolute Contraindications

- Any prior intracranial hemorrhage
- Known structural cerebral vascular lesion (eg, arteriovenous malformation)
- Known malignant intracranial neoplasm (primary or metastatic)
- Ischemic stroke within 3 months
  – **Except** acute ischemic stroke within 4.5 hours
- Suspected aortic dissection
- Active bleeding or bleeding diathesis (excluding menses)
- Significant closed head trauma or facial trauma within 3 months
- Intracranial or intraspinal surgery within 2 months
- Severe uncontrolled hypertension (unresponsive to emergency therapy)
- For streptokinase, prior treatment within the previous 6 months

## Relative Contraindications

- History of chronic, severe, poorly controlled hypertension
- Significant hypertension on presentation (systolic blood pressure greater than 180 mm Hg or diastolic blood pressure greater than 110 mm Hg)
- History of prior ischemic stroke more than 3 months
- Dementia
- Known intracranial pathology not covered in contraindications
- Traumatic or prolonged (more than 10 minutes) CPR
- Major surgery (less than 3 weeks)
- Recent (within 2 to 4 weeks) internal bleeding
- Noncompressible vascular punctures
- Pregnancy
- Active peptic ulcer
- Oral anticoagulant therapy

### Tenecteplase

- Bolus, weight adjusted
  - Less than 60 kg: Give 30 mg.
  - 60 to 69 kg: Give 35 mg.
  - 70 to 79 kg: Give 40 mg.
  - 80 to 89 kg: Give 45 mg.
  - 90 kg or more: Give 50 mg.
- Administer single IV bolus over 5 seconds.
- Incompatible with dextrose solutions.

### Reteplase, Recombinant

- Give first 10 unit IV bolus over 2 minutes.
- 30 minutes later, give second 10 unit IV bolus over 2 minutes. (Give NS flush before and after each bolus.)

*See Advanced Cardiovascular Life Support Drugs section for complete details.

## Conveying News of a Sudden Death to Family Members

- Before talking to the family, obtain as much information as possible about the patient and the circumstances surrounding the death. Be ready to refer to the patient by name.
- Call the family if they have not been notified. Explain that their loved one has been admitted to the emergency department or critical care unit and that the situation is serious. If possible, family members should be told of the death in person, not over the telephone.
- When family members arrive, ask someone to take them to a private area. Walk in, introduce yourself, and sit down. Ask if everyone is present, and have the family members introduce themselves. Address the closest relative. Maintain eye contact and position yourself at the same level as family members (ie, sitting or standing).
- Enlist the aid of a social worker or a member of the clergy if possible.
- Briefly describe the circumstances leading to the death. Summarize the sequence of events. Avoid euphemisms such as "he's passed on," "she's no longer with us," or "he's left us." Instead use the words "death," "dying," or "dead."
- Allow time for family members to process the information. Make eye contact, touch, and share

feelings with a simple phrase such as "You have my (our) sincere sympathy."
- Determine the patient's suitability for and wishes about tissue donation (use driver's license and patient records). Follow local protocols on when to discuss with family. Consent for donation should be requested by a trained individual who is not part of the care team.
- Allow as much time as necessary for questions and discussion. Review the events several times if needed.
- Allow family members the opportunity to see the patient. Prepare the family for what they will see. If equipment is still connected to the patient, tell the family. Equipment must be left in place for coroner's cases or when an autopsy is performed.
- Determine in advance what happens next and who will sign the death certificate. Physicians may impose burdens on staff and family if they fail to understand policies about death certification and disposition of the body.
- Offer to contact the patient's attending or family physician and to be available if there are further questions. Arrange for follow-up and continued support during the grieving period.

According to surveys in the United States and the United Kingdom, most family members state that they would like to be present during the attempted resuscitation of a loved one. Parents and care providers of chronically ill patients are often knowledgeable about and comfortable with medical equipment and emergency procedures. Even family members with no medical background report that it is comforting to be at the side of a loved one and say goodbye during the final moments of life. For those who choose to be at the bedside, have a designated support person with them to answer questions, clarify information, and comfort the family. Family members often do not ask if they can be present, but healthcare providers should offer the opportunity whenever possible.

Relatives and friends who are present and are provided counseling during resuscitation of a loved one report fewer incidences of posttraumatic avoidance behaviors, fewer grieving symptoms, and less intrusive imagery.

When family members are present during resuscitative efforts, sensitivity is heightened among resuscitation team members. A team member who is knowledgeable about resuscitation practices should be available to answer questions, provide comfort, and help the family during the resuscitation. Even when the resuscitation outcome is not optimal, families feel comforted to know they can be present to say goodbye, give comfort to their dying loved one, and begin the grieving process.

| Drug/Therapy | Indications/Precautions | Adult Dosage |
|---|---|---|
| **Abciximab** (ReoPro) | **Indications**<br>FDA approved for patients with planned NSTE-ACS PCI within 24 hours<br><br>**Precautions/Contraindications**<br>Binds irreversibly with platelets; platelet function recovery requires 48 hours (regeneration).<br>• Active internal bleeding or bleeding disorder in past 30 days, history of intracranial hemorrhage or other bleeding, surgical procedure or trauma within 1 month, platelet count < 150 000/mm³, hypersensitivity and concomitant use of another GP IIb/IIIa inhibitor (also see Acute Coronary Syndromes: Treatment Recommendations)<br>• Intended for use with aspirin and heparin and has been readministration may cause hypersensitivity reaction | ***Note:*** **Check package insert for current indications, doses, and duration of therapy.**<br>Optimal duration of therapy has not been established.<br><br>• **PCI:** 0.25 mg/kg IV bolus (10 to 60 minutes before procedure), then 0.125 mcg/kg per minute (to maximum of 10 mcg/min) IV infusion for 12 hours<br>• **Acute coronary syndrome (ACS) with planned PCI within 24 hours:** 0.25 mg/kg IV bolus, then 10 mcg/min IV infusion for 18 to 24 hours, concluding 1 hour after PCI |

## Administration Notes

| | |
|---|---|
| **Peripheral intravenous (IV):** | Resuscitation drugs administered via peripheral IV catheter should be followed by bolus of 20 mL IV fluid to move drug into central circulation. Then elevate extremity for 10 to 20 seconds. |
| **Intraosseous (IO):** | ACLS drugs that can be administered by IV route can be administered by IO route. |
| **Endotracheal:** | IV/IO administration is preferred because it provides more reliable drug delivery and pharmacologic effect. Drugs that can be administered by endotracheal route are noted in the table below. Optimal endotracheal doses have not yet been established. Medication delivered via endotracheal tube should be diluted in sterile water or NS to a volume of 5 to 10 mL. Provide several positive-pressure breaths after medication is instilled. |

## ACE

*(angiotensin-converting enzyme)*

### Inhibitors

**Captopril**

**Enalapril**

**Lisinopril**

**Ramipril**

### Indications

- ACE inhibitors reduce mortality and improve LV dysfunction in post-AMI patients; they help prevent adverse LV remodeling, delay progression of heart failure, and decrease sudden death and recurrent MI
- An ACE inhibitor should be administered orally within the first 24 hours after onset of AMI symptoms and continued long term if tolerated
- Clinical heart failure without hypotension in patients not responding to digitalis or diuretics
- Clinical signs of AMI with LV dysfunction
- LV ejection fraction <40%

### Precautions/Contraindications for All ACE Inhibitors

- **Contraindicated** in pregnancy (may cause fetal injury or death)
- Contraindicated in angioedema
- Hypersensitivity to ACE inhibitors
- Reduce dose in renal failure (creatinine >2.5 mg/dL in men, >2 mg/dL in women); avoid in bilateral renal artery stenosis
- Serum potassium >5 mEq/L
- Do not give if patient is hypotensive (systolic blood pressure <100 mm Hg or >30 mm Hg below baseline) or volume depleted
- Generally not started in ED; after reperfusion therapy has been completed and blood pressure has stabilized, start within 24 hours

**Approach:** ACE inhibitor therapy should start with low-dose oral administration (with possible IV doses for some preparations) and increase steadily to achieve a full dose within 24 to 48 hours.

An angiotensin receptor blocker (ARB) should be administered to patients intolerant of ACE inhibitors.

### Captopril, AMI Dose

- Start with a single dose of 6.25 mg PO
- Advance to 25 mg TID and then to 50 mg TID as tolerated

### Enalapril (IV = Enalaprilat)

- **PO:** Start with a single dose of 2.5 mg; titrate to 20 mg PO BID
- **IV:** 1.25 mg IV initial dose over 5 minutes, then 1.25 to 5 mg IV every 6 hours
- IV form is contraindicated in STEMI (risk of hypotension)

### Lisinopril, AMI Dose

- 5 mg within 24 hours after onset of symptoms, then
- 5 mg given after 24 hours, then
- 10 mg given after 48 hours, then
- 10 mg once daily

### Ramipril

Start with a single dose of 2.5 mg PO. Titrate to 5 mg PO BID as tolerated.

| Drug/Therapy | Indications/Precautions | Adult Dosage |
|---|---|---|
| **Adenosine** | **Indications** <br> • First drug for most forms of stable narrow-complex SVT; effective in terminating those due to reentry involving AV node or sinus node <br> • May consider for unstable narrow-complex reentry tachycardia while preparations are made for cardioversion <br> • Regular and monomorphic wide-complex tachycardia, thought to be or previously defined to be reentry SVT <br> • Does not convert atrial fibrillation, atrial flutter, or VT <br> • Diagnostic maneuver: stable narrow-complex SVT <br><br> **Precautions/Contraindications** <br> • Contraindicated in poison/drug-induced tachycardia or second- or third-degree heart block <br> • Transient side effects include flushing, chest pain or tightness, brief periods of asystole or bradycardia, ventricular ectopy <br> • Less effective (larger doses may be required) in patients taking theophylline or caffeine <br> • Reduce initial dose to 3 mg in patients receiving dipyridamole or carbamazepine, in heart transplant patients, or if given by central venous access <br> • If administered for irregular, polymorphic wide-complex tachycardia/VT, may cause deterioration (including hypotension) <br> • Transient periods of sinus bradycardia and ventricular ectopy are common after termination of SVT <br> • Safe and effective in pregnancy | **IV Rapid Push** <br> • Place patient in mild reverse Trendelenburg position before administration of drug <br> • Initial bolus of 6 mg given *rapidly* over 1 to 3 seconds followed by NS bolus of 20 mL; then elevate the extremity <br> • A second dose (12 mg) can be given in 1 to 2 minutes if needed <br><br> **Injection Technique** <br> • Record rhythm strip during administration <br> • Draw up adenosine dose in one syringe and flush in another; attach both syringes to the same or immediately adjacent IV injection ports nearest patient, with adenosine closest to patient port <br> • Clamp IV tubing above injection port <br> • Push IV adenosine as quickly as possible (1 to 3 seconds) <br> • While maintaining pressure on adenosine plunger, push NS flush as rapidly as possible after adenosine <br> • Unclamp IV tubing |

**Alteplase, Recombinant**
(Activase)
**Tissue Plasminogen Activator**
(alteplase)
(see *Fibrinolytic Agents*)

---

**Amiodarone**

Amiodarone is a complex drug with effects on sodium, potassium, and calcium channels as well as α- and β-adrenergic blocking properties. Patients must be hospitalized while the loading doses of amiodarone are administered. Amiodarone should be prescribed only by physicians who are experienced in the treatment of life-threatening arrhythmias, are thoroughly familiar with amiodarone's risks and benefits, and have access to laboratory facilities capable of adequately monitoring the effectiveness and side effects of amiodarone treatment.

Indications

Because its use is associated with toxicity, amiodarone is indicated for use in patients with life-threatening arrhythmias when administered with appropriate monitoring:

**VF/pVT Cardiac Arrest Unresponsive to CPR, Shock, and Vasopressor**
- First dose: 300 mg IV/IO push
- Second dose (if needed): 150 mg IV/IO push

**Life-Threatening Arrhythmias**
**Maximum cumulative dose:** 2.2 g IV over 24 hours. May be administered as follows
- **Rapid infusion**: 150 mg IV over first 10 minutes (15 mg/min). May repeat rapid infusion (150 mg IV) every 10 minutes as needed
- **Slow infusion**: 360 mg IV over 6 hours (1 mg/min)
- **Maintenance infusion**: 540 mg IV over 18 hours (0.5 mg/min)

*(continued)*

| Drug/Therapy | Indications/Precautions | Adult Dosage |
|---|---|---|
| **Amiodarone** *(continued)* | • VF/pVT unresponsive to shock delivery, CPR, and a vasopressor<br>• Recurrent, hemodynamically unstable VT<br><br>With expert consultation, amiodarone may be used for treatment of some atrial and ventricular arrhythmias.<br><br>***Caution: Multiple complex drug interactions*** | **Precautions**<br>• Rapid infusion may lead to hypotension<br>• With multiple dosing, cumulative doses >2.2 g over 24 hours are associated with significant hypotension in clinical trials<br>• Do not administer with other drugs that prolong QT interval (eg, procainamide)<br>• Terminal elimination is extremely long (half-life lasts up to 40 days) |
| **Aspirin** | **Indications**<br>• Administer to all patients with ACS, particularly reperfusion candidates, unless hypersensitive to aspirin<br>• Blocks formation of thromboxane $A_2$, which causes platelets to aggregate and arteries to constrict; this reduces overall ACS mortality, reinfarction, and nonfatal stroke<br>• Any person with symptoms ("pressure," "heavy weight," "squeezing," "crushing") suggestive of ischemic pain<br>**Precautions/Contraindications**<br>• Relatively contraindicated in patients with active ulcer disease or asthma<br>• Contraindicated in patients with known hypersensitivity to aspirin | • Chew 162 to 325 mg tablet as soon as possible<br>• May use rectal suppository (300 mg) for patients who cannot take orally |

## Atenolol
*(see β-Blockers)*

## Atropine Sulfate

Can be given via endotracheal tube

### Indications

- First drug for symptomatic sinus bradycardia
- May be beneficial in presence of AV nodal block; **not likely to be effective for type II second-degree or third-degree AV block or a block in non-nodal tissue**
- Routine use during PEA or asystole is unlikely to have a therapeutic benefit
- Organophosphate (eg, nerve agent) poisoning: extremely large doses may be needed

### Precautions

- Use with caution in presence of myocardial ischemia and hypoxia. Increases myocardial oxygen demand
- Unlikely to be effective for hypothermic bradycardia
- May not be effective for infranodal (type II) AV block and new third-degree block with wide QRS complexes (in these patients may cause paradoxical slowing; be prepared to pace or give catecholamines)
- Do not give to heart transplant patients

### Bradycardia (With or Without ACS)

- 1 mg IV every 3 to 5 minutes as needed, not to exceed total dose of 0.04 mg/kg (total 3 mg)

### Organophosphate Poisoning

Extremely large doses (2 to 4 mg or higher) may be needed

| Drug/Therapy | Indications/Precautions | Adult Dosage |
|---|---|---|
| **β-Blockers**<br><br>Metoprolol Tartrate<br><br>Atenolol<br><br>Propranolol<br><br>Esmolol<br><br>Labetalol<br><br>Carvedilol | **Indications (Apply to All β-Blockers)**<br>• Administer to all patients with suspected myocardial infarction and unstable angina in the absence of contraindications; these are effective antianginal agents and can reduce incidence of VF<br>• Useful as an adjunctive agent with fibrinolytic therapy; may reduce nonfatal reinfarction and recurrent ischemia<br>• To convert to normal sinus rhythm or to slow ventricular response (or both) in supraventricular tachyarrhythmias (reentry SVT, atrial fibrillation, or atrial flutter); β-blockers are second-line agents after adenosine<br>• To reduce myocardial ischemia and damage in AMI patients with elevated heart rate, blood pressure, or both<br>• Labetalol recommended for emergency antihypertensive therapy for hemorrhagic and acute ischemic stroke<br><br>**Precautions/Contraindications**<br>**(Apply to All β-Blockers Unless Noted)**<br>• Early aggressive β-blockade may be hazardous in hemodynamically unstable patients | **Metoprolol Tartrate (AMI Regimen)**<br>• 25 to 50 mg every 6 to 12 hours PO; then transition over next 2 to 3 days to twice-daily dosing of metoprolol tartrate or to daily metoprolol succinate; titrate to daily dose of 200 mg as tolerated<br><br>**Atenolol (AMI Regimen)**<br>• 5 mg IV every 5 minutes as tolerated up to 3 doses; titrate to heart rate and blood pressure<br>• 5 mg IV over 5 minutes<br>• Wait 10 minutes, then give second dose of 5 mg IV over 5 minutes<br>• In 10 minutes, if tolerated well, begin oral regimen with 50 mg PO; titrate to effect<br><br>**Propranolol (for SVT)**<br>0.5 to 1 mg over 1 minute, repeated as needed up to a total dose of 0.1 mg/kg<br><br>**Esmolol**<br>0.5 mg/kg (500 mcg/kg) over 1 minute, followed by 0.05 mg/kg (50 mcg/kg) per minute infusion; maximum: 0.3 mg/kg (300 mcg/kg) per minute |

*(continued)*

**β-Blockers**
(continued)

- Do not give to patients with STEMI if any of the following are present:
  - Signs of heart failure
  - Low cardiac output
  - Increased risk for cardiogenic shock
- Relative contraindications include PR interval >0.24 second, second- or third-degree heart block, active asthma, reactive airway disease, severe bradycardia, systolic blood pressure <100 mm Hg
- Concurrent IV administration with IV calcium channel blocking agents like verapamil or diltiazem can cause severe hypotension and bradycardia/heart block
- Monitor cardiac and pulmonary status during administration
- Propranolol is contraindicated and other β-blockers relatively contraindicated in cocaine-induced ACS

- If inadequate response after 5 minutes, may repeat 0.5 mg/kg (500 mcg/kg) bolus and then titrate infusion up to 0.2 mg/kg (200 mcg/kg) per minute; higher doses unlikely to be beneficial
- Has a short half-life (2 to 9 minutes)

**Labetalol**
- 10 mg IV push over 1 to 2 minutes
- May repeat or double every 10 minutes to a maximum dose of 150 mg, or give initial dose as a bolus, then start infusion at 2 to 8 mg/min

**Carvedilol**
6.25 mg twice daily; titrate to 25 mg twice daily as tolerated

---

**Bivalirudin**

**Indications**
This is a direct thrombin inhibitor for use in ACS
- Useful as an anticoagulant with or without prior treatment with UFH in STEMI or NSTE-ACS patients undergoing PCI
- Preferred over UFH with GP IIb/IIIa inhibitors in patients undergoing PCI who are at high risk of bleeding

**Precautions**
Reduce infusion to 1 mg/kg per hour with estimated creatinine clearance <30 mL/min

**STEMI**
- 0.75 mg/kg IV bolus, then 1.75 mg/kg per hour infusion
- An additional bolus of 0.3 mg/kg may be given if needed

**NSTE-ACS**
- 0.1 mg/kg IV loading dose followed by 0.25 mg/kg per hour
- Only for patients managed with an early invasive strategy
- Continued until diagnostic angiography or PCI

| Drug/Therapy | Indications/Precautions | Adult Dosage |
|---|---|---|
| **Calcium Chloride**<br>10% solution is<br>100 mg/mL | **Indications**<br>• Known or suspected hyperkalemia (eg, renal failure)<br>• Ionized hypocalcemia (eg, after multiple blood transfusions)<br>• As an antidote for toxic effects (hypotension and arrhythmias) from calcium channel blocker overdose or β-blocker overdose<br><br>**Precautions**<br>• Do not use routinely in cardiac arrest<br>• Do not mix with sodium bicarbonate | **Typical Dose**<br>• 500 mg to 1000 mg (5 to 10 mL of a 10% solution) IV for hyperkalemia and calcium channel blocker overdose; may be repeated as needed<br>• *Note:* Comparable dose of 10% calcium gluconate is 15 to 30 mL. |
| **Cangrelor**<br>(Kengreal)<br>(see *P2Y₁₂ Receptor Blockers*) | | |
| **Captopril**<br>(see *ACE Inhibitors*) | | |

## Clevidipine
**Calcium channel blocker**

### Indications
- Hypertensive emergencies
- Decrease blood pressure to ≤185/110 mm Hg before administration of fibrinolytic therapy

### Precautions/Contraindications
- Avoid rapid decrease in blood pressure
- Reflex tachycardia or increased angina may occur in patients with extensive coronary disease
- Avoid use in patients with severe aortic stenosis
- Lipid emulsion
  - Do not dilute IV solution; maintain aseptic technique and discard tubing and unused drug after 12 hours
  - Hypertriglyceridemia may result from high dose or extended infusions
  - Do not use in patients with soy, soybean, or egg allergy or in patients with acute pancreatitis
- May be confused with other lipid emulsions such as propofol

### Acute Hypertension Emergencies
Initial infusion rate 1 to 2 mg per hour IV, titrate by doubling the dose every 2 to 5 minutes until desired blood pressure reached; maximum 21 mg per hour

## Clopidogrel
(Plavix)
(see *P2Y₁₂ Receptor Blockers*)

| Drug/Therapy | Indications/Precautions | Adult Dosage |
|---|---|---|
| **Digoxin**<br><br>0.25 mg/mL or<br>0.1 mg/mL; supplied in<br>1 or 2 mL ampule<br>(totals = 0.1–0.5 mg) | **Indications (May Be of Limited Use)**<br>• To slow ventricular response in atrial fibrillation or atrial flutter<br>• Alternative drug for reentry SVT<br><br>**Precautions**<br>• Toxic effects are common and are frequently associated with serious arrhythmias<br>• Avoid electrical cardioversion if patient is receiving digoxin unless condition is life threatening; use lower dose (10–20 J) | **IV Administration**<br>• Loading doses: 0.004–0.006 mg/kg (4–6 mcg/kg) initially over 5 minutes; second and third boluses of 0.002–0.003 mg/kg (2–3 mcg/kg) to follow at 4- to 8-hour intervals (total loading dose 8–12 mcg/kg divided over 8–16 hours)<br>• Check digoxin levels no sooner than 4 hours after IV dose; no sooner than 6 hours after oral dose<br>• Monitor heart rate and ECG<br>• Maintenance dose is affected by body mass and renal function<br>• **Caution: Amiodarone interaction;** reduce digoxin dose by 50% when used with amiodarone |
| **Digoxin-Specific Antibody Therapy**<br><br>Digibind (38 mg) or<br>DigiFab (40 mg)<br>(each vial binds about<br>0.5 mg digoxin) | **Indications**<br>Digoxin toxicity with the following:<br>• Life-threatening arrhythmias<br>• Shock or congestive heart failure<br>• Hyperkalemia (potassium level > 5 mEq/L)<br>• Steady-state serum levels > 10–15 ng/mL for symptomatic patients<br><br>**Precautions**<br>Serum digoxin levels rise after digoxin antibody therapy and should not be used to guide continuing therapy. | **Chronic Intoxication**<br>3–5 vials may be effective.<br><br>**Acute Overdose**<br>• IV dose varies according to amount of digoxin ingested; see ACLS Toxicology<br>• Average dose is 10 vials; may require up to 20 vials<br>• See package insert for details |

## Diltiazem

### Indications

- To control ventricular rate in atrial fibrillation and atrial flutter; may terminate reentrant arrhythmias that require AV nodal conduction for their continuation
- Use after adenosine to treat refractory reentry SVT in patients with narrow QRS complex and adequate blood pressure

### Precautions

- Do not use calcium channel blockers for wide-QRS tachycardias of uncertain origin or for poison/drug-induced tachycardia
- Avoid calcium channel blockers in patients with Wolff-Parkinson-White syndrome plus rapid atrial fibrillation or flutter, in patients with sick sinus syndrome, or in patients with AV block without a pacemaker
- *Caution*: Blood pressure may drop from peripheral vasodilation (greater drop with verapamil than with diltiazem)
- Concurrent IV administration with IV β-blockers may produce severe hypotension; use with extreme caution in patients receiving oral β-blockers

### Acute Rate Control

- 15-20 mg (0.25 mg/kg) IV over 2 minutes
- May give another IV dose in 15 minutes at 20-25 mg (0.35 mg/kg) over 2 minutes

### Maintenance Infusion

5-15 mg per hour, titrated to physiologically appropriate heart rate (can dilute in $D_5W$ or NS)

| Drug/Therapy | Indications/Precautions | Adult Dosage |
|---|---|---|
| **Dobutamine**<br>IV infusion | **Indications**<br>Consider for pump problems (congestive heart failure, pulmonary congestion) with systolic blood pressure of 70-100 mm Hg and no signs of shock<br><br>**Precautions/Contraindications**<br>• Contraindication: Suspected or known poison/drug-induced shock<br>• Avoid with systolic blood pressure <100 mm Hg and signs of shock<br>• May cause tachyarrhythmias, fluctuations in blood pressure, headache, and nausea<br>• Do not mix with sodium bicarbonate<br>• Increases in heart rate of more than 10% may induce or exacerbate myocardial ischemia | **IV Administration**<br>• Usual infusion rate is 2-20 mcg/kg per minute<br>• Hemodynamic monitoring is recommended for optimal use<br>• Elderly patients may have a significantly decreased response |

## Dopamine
IV infusion

**Indications**
- Second-line drug for symptomatic bradycardia (after atropine)
- Use for hypotension (systolic blood pressure ≤70-100 mm Hg) with signs and symptoms of shock

**Precautions**
- Correct hypovolemia with volume replacement before initiating dopamine
- Use with caution in cardiogenic shock with accompanying congestive heart failure
- May cause tachyarrhythmias, excessive vasoconstriction
- Do not mix with sodium bicarbonate

**IV Administration**
- Usual infusion rate is 5-20 mcg/kg per minute
- Titrate to patient response; taper slowly

---

## Enalapril
(*see ACE Inhibitors*)

| Drug/Therapy | Indications/Precautions | Adult Dosage |
|---|---|---|
| **Epinephrine**<br><br>Can be given via endotracheal tube<br><br>Available in 0.1 mg/mL and 1 mg/mL concentrations | **Indications**<br>- **Cardiac arrest:** VF, pVT, asystole, PEA<br>- **Symptomatic bradycardia:** Can be considered after atropine to dopamine as an alternative infusion<br>- **Severe hypotension:** Can be used when pacing and atropine fail, when hypotension accompanies bradycardia, or with phosphodiesterase enzyme inhibitor<br>- **Anaphylaxis, severe allergic reactions:** Combine with large fluid volume, corticosteroids, antihistamines<br><br>**Precautions**<br>- Raising blood pressure and increasing heart rate may cause myocardial ischemia, angina, and increased myocardial oxygen demand<br>- High doses do not improve survival or neurologic outcome and may contribute to postresuscitation myocardial dysfunction<br>- Higher doses *may* be required to treat poisoning/drug-induced shock | **Cardiac Arrest**<br>- **IV/IO dose:** 1 mg (10 mL of 0.1 mg/mL solution) administered every 3-5 minutes during resuscitation; follow each dose with 20 mL flush, elevate arm for 10-20 seconds after dose<br>- **Higher dose:** Higher doses (up to 0.2 mg/kg) may be used for specific indications (β-blocker or calcium channel blocker overdose)<br>- **Continuous infusion:** Initial rate: 0.1-0.5 mcg/kg per minute (for 70-kg patient: 7-35 mcg/min); titrate to response<br>- **Endotracheal route:** 2-2.5 mg diluted in 10 mL NS<br><br>**Profound Bradycardia or Hypotension**<br>2-10 mcg/min infusion; titrate to patient response |

## Eptifibatide

### Indications
For high-risk NSTE-ACS and patients undergoing PCI

### Actions/Precautions
Platelet function recovers within 4-8 hours after discontinuation

### Contraindications
Active internal bleeding or bleeding disorder in past 30 days, history of intracranial hemorrhage or other bleeding, surgical procedure or trauma within 1 month, platelet count <150 000/mm$^3$, hypersensitivity and concomitant use of another GP IIb/IIIa inhibitor (also see Acute Coronary Syndromes: Treatment Recommendations)

***Note:* Check package insert for current indications, doses, and duration of therapy.** Optimal duration of therapy has not been established.
- **PCI**: 180 mcg/kg IV bolus over 1-2 minutes, then begin 2 mcg/kg per minute IV infusion, then repeat bolus in 10 minutes
- Maximum dose (121-kg patient) for PCI: 22.6 mg bolus; 15 mg per hour infusion
- Infusion duration 18-24 hours after PCI
- Reduce rate of infusion by 50% if creatinine clearance <50 mL/min

## Esmolol
(*see β-Blockers*)

| Drug/Therapy | Indications/Precautions | Adult Dosage |
| --- | --- | --- |
| **Fibrinolytic Agents**<br><br>**Alteplase, Recombinant** (Activase)<br>**Reteplase, Recombinant** (Retavase)<br>**Tenecteplase** (TNKase) | **Indications**<br>**Cardiac arrest:** Insufficient evidence to recommend routine use<br>**AMI in adults:**<br>• ST elevation (threshold values: J-point elevation of 2 mm in leads $V_2$ and $V_3$* and 1 mm in all other leads) or new or presumably new LBBB<br>• In context of signs and symptoms of AMI<br>• Time from onset of symptoms ≤12 hours<br>• See Acute Coronary Syndromes: Fibrinolytic Therapy for guidance on use of fibrinolytics in patients with STEMI<br>*Threshold value of 2.5 mm in men <40 years; 1.5 mm in all women<br>**Acute ischemic stroke:**<br>(Alteplase is the only fibrinolytic agent approved for acute ischemic stroke.)<br>• Sudden onset of focal neurologic deficits or alterations in consciousness (eg, facial droop, arm drift, abnormal speech) | For all 3 agents, insert 2 peripheral IV lines; use 1 line exclusively for fibrinolytic administration<br>**Alteplase, Recombinant (rtPA)**<br>50- and 100-mg vials reconstituted with sterile water to 1 mg/mL<br><br>Recommended total dose is based on patient's weight<br>**STEMI:**<br>• Accelerated infusion (1.5 hours)<br>  – Give 15 mg IV bolus<br>  – Then 0.75 mg/kg over next 30 minutes (not to exceed 50 mg)<br>  – Then 0.5 mg/kg over 60 minutes (not to exceed 35 mg)<br>  – Maximum total dose: 100 mg<br>**Acute ischemic stroke:**<br>• Give 0.9 mg/kg (maximum 90 mg) IV, infused over 60 minutes<br>• Give 10% of total dose as an initial IV bolus over 1 minute<br>• Give remaining 90% of total dose IV over next 60 minutes |

(continued)

## Fibrinolytic Agents
*(continued)*

- See Use of IV Alteplase for Acute Ischemic Stroke: Inclusion and Exclusion Characteristics for guidance on which patients can be treated with alteplase based on time of symptom onset

**Precautions and Possible Exclusion Criteria for AMI in Adults/Acute Ischemic Stroke**

- For AMI in adults, see Acute Coronary Syndromes: Fibrinolytic Therapy for indications, precautions, and contraindications
- For acute ischemic stroke, see Use of IV Alteplase for Acute Ischemic Stroke: Inclusion and Exclusion Characteristics for indications, precautions, and contraindications

**Reteplase, Recombinant (STEMI)**

10-unit vials reconstituted with sterile water to 1 unit/mL

- Give first 10-unit IV bolus over 2 minutes
- 30 minutes later, give second 10-unit IV bolus over 2 minutes (give NS flush before and after each bolus)

**Tenecteplase (STEMI)**

- Administer single IV bolus over 5 seconds
- Incompatible with dextrose solutions

**STEMI**

50-mg vial reconstituted with sterile water

- Bolus, weight adjusted
  - <60 kg: Give 30 mg
  - 60-69 kg: Give 35 mg
  - 70-79 kg: Give 40 mg
  - 80-89 kg: Give 45 mg
  - ≥90 kg: Give 50 mg

| Drug/Therapy | Indications/Precautions | Adult Dosage |
|---|---|---|
| **Flumazenil** | **Indications** | |
| | Reverse respiratory depression and sedative effects from pure benzodiazepine overdose | **First Dose** |
| | | 0.2 mg IV over 15 seconds |
| | **Precautions** | **Second Dose** |
| | • Effects may not outlast effect of benzodiazepines | 0.3 mg IV over 30 seconds; if no adequate response, give third dose |
| | • Monitor for recurrent respiratory depression | **Third Dose** |
| | • Do not use in suspected tricyclic overdose | 0.5 mg IV given over 30 seconds; if no adequate response, repeat once every minute until adequate response or a total of 3 mg is given |
| | • Do not use in seizure-prone patients, chronic benzodiazepine users, or alcoholics | |
| | • Do not use in unknown drug or mixed drug overdose with drugs known to cause seizures (tricyclic antidepressants, cocaine, amphetamines, etc) | |

## Fondaparinux
(Arixtra)

### Indications
- For use in ACS
- To inhibit thrombin generation by factor Xa inhibition
- May be used for anticoagulation in patients with history of heparin-induced thrombocytopenia

### Precautions/Contraindications
- Hemorrhage may complicate therapy
- Contraindicated in patients with creatinine clearance <30 mL/min; use with caution in patients with creatinine clearance 30-50 mL/min

**Increased risk of catheter thrombosis in patients undergoing PCI; coadministration of unfractionated heparin required**

### STEMI Protocol
Initial dose 2.5 mg IV bolus followed by 2.5 mg subcutaneously every 24 hours for up to 8 days

### NSTE-ACS Protocol
2.5 mg subcutaneously every 24 hours

---

## Furosemide

### Indications
- For adjuvant therapy of acute pulmonary edema in patients with SBP >90-100 mm Hg (without signs and symptoms of shock)
- Hypertensive emergencies

### Precautions
Dehydration, hypovolemia, hypotension, hypokalemia, or other electrolyte imbalance may occur.

### IV Administration
- 0.5-1 mg/kg given over 1-2 minutes
- If no response, double dose to 2 mg/kg, given slowly over 1-2 minutes
- For new-onset pulmonary edema with hypovolemia: <0.5 mg/kg

# Advanced Cardiovascular Life Support Drugs

| Drug/Therapy | Indications/Precautions | Adult Dosage |
|---|---|---|
| **Glucagon**<br>Powdered in 1-mg vials<br><br>Reconstitute with provided solution | **Indications**<br>Adjuvant treatment of toxic effects of calcium channel blocker or β-blocker.<br><br>**Precautions**<br>May cause vomiting, hyperglycemia | **IV Infusion**<br>3-10 mg IV slowly over 3-5 minutes, followed by infusion of 3-5 mg per hour |
| *Glycoprotein IIb/IIIa Inhibitors*<br><br>**Abciximab**<br>(ReoPro)<br>**Eptifibatide**<br>(Integrilin)<br>**Tirofiban**<br>(Aggrastat)<br>(See individual drug listings for indications, precautions, and contraindications.) | | |

## Heparin, unfractionated
(UFH)

Concentrations range from 1000 to 40 000 units/mL

**Indications**
- Adjunct therapy in AMI
- Begin heparin with fibrin-specific lytics (eg, alteplase, reteplase, tenecteplase)

**Precautions/Contraindications**
- Same contraindications as for fibrinolytic therapy: active bleeding; recent intracranial, intraspinal, or eye surgery; severe hypertension; bleeding disorders; gastrointestinal bleeding
- Doses and laboratory targets appropriate when used with fibrinolytic therapy
- Do not use if platelet count is or falls below <100 000/mm$^3$ or with history of heparin-induced thrombocytopenia; for these patients, consider direct antithrombins

**UFH IV Infusion—STEMI**
- Initial bolus 60 units/kg (maximum bolus: 4000 units)
- Continue 12 units/kg per hour, round to the nearest 50 units (maximum initial rate: 1000 units per hour)
- Adjust to maintain aPTT 1.5-2 times the control values for 48 hours or until angiography
- Check initial aPTT at 3 hours, then every 6 hours until stable, then daily
- Follow institutional heparin protocol
- Platelet count daily

**UFH IV Infusion—NSTE-ACS**
- Initial bolus 60 units/kg; maximum: 4000 units
- 12 units/kg per hour; maximum initial rate: 1000 units per hour
- Follow institutional protocol (see Heparin in ACS section)

| Drug/Therapy | Indications/Precautions | Adult Dosage |
|---|---|---|
| **Heparin, Low Molecular Weight (LMWH)** | **Indications**<br>For use in ACS, specifically patients with NSTE-ACS; these drugs inhibit thrombin generation by factor Xa inhibition and also inhibit thrombin indirectly by formation of a complex with antithrombin III; these drugs are not neutralized by heparin-binding proteins<br><br>**Precautions**<br>• Hemorrhage may complicate any therapy with LMWH; contraindicated in presence of hypersensitivity to heparin or pork products or history of sensitivity to drug; use LMWH with extreme caution in patients with type II heparin-induced thrombocytopenia<br>• Adjust dose for renal insufficiency<br>• Contraindicated if platelet count < 100 000/mm³; for these patients, consider direct antithrombins | **STEMI Protocol**<br>• Enoxaparin<br>  – Age <75 years, normal creatinine clearance: Initial bolus 30 mg IV with second bolus 15 minutes later of 1 mg/kg subcutaneously; repeat every 12 hours (maximum 100 mg/dose for first 2 doses)<br>  – Age ≥75 years: Eliminate initial IV bolus; give 0.75 mg/kg subcutaneously every 12 hours (maximum 75 mg/dose for first 2 doses)<br>  – If creatinine clearance <30 mL/min, give 1 mg/kg subcutaneously every 24 hours<br><br>**NSTE-ACS Protocol**<br>Enoxaparin: Loading dose 30 mg IV bolus; maintenance dose 1 mg/kg subcutaneously every 12 hours; if creatinine clearance <30 mL/min, give every 24 hours |

## Ibutilide

Intervention of choice is DC cardioversion

### Indications

Treatment of supraventricular arrhythmias, including atrial fibrillation and atrial flutter when duration ≤48 hours; short duration of action; effective for the conversion of atrial fibrillation or flutter of relatively brief duration

### Precautions/Contraindications

Contraindication: Do not give to patients with $QT_c$ >440 milliseconds. Ventricular arrhythmias develop in approximately 2%-5% of patients (polymorphic VT, including torsades de pointes). *Monitor ECG continuously for arrhythmias during administration and for 4-6 hours after administration with defibrillator nearby.* Patients with significantly impaired LV function are at highest risk for arrhythmias.

### Dose for Adults ≥60 kg

1 mg (10 mL) administered IV (diluted or undiluted) over 10 minutes; a second dose may be administered at the same rate 10 minutes later

### Dose for Adults <60 kg

0.01 mg/kg initial IV dose administered over 10 minutes

| Drug/Therapy | Indications/Precautions | Adult Dosage |
|---|---|---|
| **Isoproterenol**<br>IV infusion | **Indications**<br>• *Use cautiously as temporizing measure if external pacer is not available for treatment of symptomatic bradycardia*<br>• Refractory torsades de pointes unresponsive to magnesium sulfate<br>• *Temporary* control of bradycardia in heart transplant patients (denervated heart unresponsive to atropine)<br>• Poisoning from β-blockers<br>**Precautions**<br>• Do not use for treatment of cardiac arrest<br>• Increases myocardial oxygen requirements, which may increase myocardial ischemia<br>• Do not give with epinephrine; can cause VF/pVT<br>• Do not give to patients with poisoning/drug-induced shock (except for β-blocker poisoning)<br>• May use higher doses for β-blocker poisoning | **IV Administration**<br>• Infuse at 2-10 mcg/min<br>• Titrate to adequate heart rate<br>• In torsades de pointes, titrate to increase heart rate until VT is suppressed |
| **Labetalol**<br>(see *β-Blockers*) | | |

## Lidocaine

Can be given via endotracheal tube

### Indications

- Alternative to amiodarone in cardiac arrest from VF/pVT
- Stable monomorphic VT with preserved ventricular function
- Stable polymorphic VT with normal baseline QT interval and preserved LV function when ischemia is treated and electrolyte balance is corrected
- Can be used for stable polymorphic VT with baseline QT-interval prolongation if torsades suspected

### Precautions/Contraindications

- Contraindication: Prophylactic use in AMI is contraindicated
- Reduce maintenance dose (not loading dose) in presence of impaired liver function or LV dysfunction
- Discontinue infusion immediately if signs of toxicity develop

### Cardiac Arrest From VF/pVT

- Initial dose: 1-1.5 mg/kg IV/IO
- For refractory VF, may give additional 0.5-0.75 mg/kg IV push and repeat in 5-10 minutes; maximum 3 doses or total of 3 mg/kg

### Perfusing Arrhythmia

For stable VT, wide-complex tachycardia of uncertain type, significant ectopy:

- Doses ranging from 0.5-0.75 mg/kg and up to 1-1.5 mg/kg may be used
- Repeat 0.5-0.75 mg/kg every 5-10 minutes; maximum total dose: 3 mg/kg

### Maintenance Infusion

1-4 mg/min (30-50 mcg/kg per minute)

---

## Lisinopril
(see **ACE Inhibitors**)

# Advanced Cardiovascular Life Support Drugs

| Drug/Therapy | Indications/Precautions | Adult Dosage |
|---|---|---|
| **Magnesium Sulfate** | **Indications**<br>• Recommended for use in cardiac arrest only if torsades de pointes or suspected hypomagnesemia is present<br>• Life-threatening ventricular arrhythmias due to digitalis toxicity<br>• Routine administration in hospitalized patients with AMI is not recommended<br><br>**Precautions**<br>• Occasional fall in blood pressure with rapid administration<br>• Use with caution if renal failure is present | **Cardiac Arrest (Due to Hypomagnesemia or Torsades de Pointes)**<br>• 1-2 g (2-4 mL of a 50% solution diluted in 10 mL [eg, normal saline] given IV/IO)<br><br>**Torsades de Pointes With a Pulse or AMI With Hypomagnesemia**<br>• Loading dose of 1-2 g mixed in 50-100 mL of diluent (eg, D$_5$W, normal saline) over 5-60 minutes IV<br>• Follow with 0.5-1 g per hour IV (titrate to control torsades) |
| **Mannitol**<br><br>Strengths: 5%, 10%, 15%, 20%, and 25% | **Indications**<br>Increased intracranial pressure in management of neurologic emergencies<br><br>**Precautions**<br>• Monitor fluid status and serum osmolality (not to exceed 310 mOsm/kg)<br>• Caution in renal failure because fluid overload may result | **IV Administration**<br>• Administer 0.5-1 g/kg over 5-10 minutes through in-line filter<br>• Additional doses of 0.25-2 g/kg can be given every 4-6 hours as needed<br>• Use with support of oxygenation and ventilation |
| **Metoprolol Tartrate** (see *β-Blockers*) | | |

## Milrinone

### Indications
Myocardial dysfunction and increased systemic or pulmonary vascular resistance, including
- Congestive heart failure in postoperative cardiovascular surgical patients
- Shock with high systemic vascular resistance

### Precautions
May produce nausea, vomiting, hypotension, particularly in volume-depleted patients; drug may accumulate in renal failure and in patients with low cardiac output; reduce dose in renal failure

### Loading Dose
50 mcg/kg over 10 minutes IV loading dose

### IV Infusion
- 0.375-0.75 mcg/kg per minute
- Hemodynamic monitoring required
- Reduce dose in renal impairment

---

## Morphine Sulfate

### Indications
- Chest pain with ACS unresponsive to nitrates
- Acute cardiogenic pulmonary edema (if blood pressure is adequate)

### Precautions
- Administer slowly and titrate to effect
- May cause respiratory depression
- Causes hypotension in volume-depleted patients
- Use with caution in RV infarction
- May reverse with naloxone (0.04-2 mg IV)

### IV Administration
- STEMI: Give 2-4 mg IV; may give additional doses of 2-8 mg IV at 5- to 15-minute intervals; analgesic of choice
- NSTE-ACS: Give 1-5 mg IV only if symptoms not relieved by nitrates or if symptoms recur; use with caution

| Drug/Therapy | Indications/Precautions | Adult Dosage |
|---|---|---|

**Naloxone Hydrochloride**

Can be given via endotracheal tube

**Indications**

Respiratory and neurologic depression due to opiate intoxication unresponsive to oxygen and support of ventilation

**Precautions**

- May cause severe opiate withdrawal, including hypertensive crisis and pulmonary edema when given in large doses (titration of small doses recommended)
- Half-life shorter than narcotics; repeat dosing may be needed
- Monitor for recurrent respiratory depression
- Rare anaphylactic reactions have been reported
- Assist ventilation before naloxone administration; avoid sympathetic stimulation
- Avoid in meperidine-induced seizures

**Administration**

- Typical IV dose 0.04-0.4 mg; titrate until ventilation adequate
- Use higher doses for complete narcotic reversal
- Can administer up to 6-10 mg over short period (<10 minutes)
- If total reversal is not required (eg, respiratory depression from sedation), smaller doses of 0.04 mg repeated every 2-3 minutes may be used
- For chronic opioid-addicted patients, use smaller dose and titrate slowly

**Opioid-Associated Life-Threatening Emergencies**

- **IM or IV:** 0.04-0.4 mg, repeated every 2-3 minutes if necessary
- **Intranasal:** 2 mg, repeated every 3-5 minutes if necessary

## Nicardipine

(Cardene)

Calcium channel blocker

**Indications**
- Hypertensive emergencies
- Decrease blood pressure to ≤185/110 mm Hg before administration of fibrinolytic therapy

**Precautions/Contraindications**
- Avoid rapid decrease in blood pressure
- Reflex tachycardia or increased angina may occur in patients with extensive coronary disease
- Avoid use in patients with severe aortic stenosis
- Do not mix with sodium bicarbonate or Ringer's lactate solution

**Acute Hypertension Emergencies**
- Initial infusion rate 5 mg per hour; may increase by 2.5 mg per hour every 5-15 minutes to maximum of 15 mg per hour
- Decrease infusion rate to 3 mg per hour once desired blood pressure reached

---

## Nitroglycerin

Available in IV form, sublingual tablets, and aerosol spray

**Indications**
- Initial antianginal for suspected ischemic pain
- For initial 24-48 hours in patients with *AMI and CHF*, large anterior wall infarction, persistent or recurrent ischemia, or hypertension
- Continued use (beyond 48 hours) for patients with recurrent angina or persistent pulmonary congestion (nitrate-free interval recommended)
- Hypertensive urgency with ACS

**IV Administration**
- **IV bolus**: 12.5-25 mcg (if no SL or spray given)
- **Infusion**: Begin at 10 mcg/min. Titrate to effect; increase by 10 mcg/min every 3-5 minutes until desired effect. Ceiling dose of 200 mcg/min commonly used
  - Route of choice for emergencies

*(continued)*

# Advanced Cardiovascular Life Support Drugs

| Drug/Therapy | Indications/Precautions | Adult Dosage |
|---|---|---|
| Nitroglycerin *(continued)* | **Contraindications** • Hypotension (systolic blood pressure <90 mm Hg or ≥30 mm Hg below baseline) • Severe bradycardia (<50/min) or tachycardia (>100/min) • RV infarction • Use of phosphodiesterase inhibitors for erectile dysfunction (eg, sildenafil and vardenafil within 24 hours; tadalafil within 48 hours)<br><br>**Precautions** • Generally, with evidence of AMI and normotension, do not reduce systolic blood pressure to <110 mm Hg; if patient is hypertensive, do not decrease mean arterial pressure (MAP) by <25% (from initial MAP) • Do not mix with other drugs • Patient should sit or lie down when receiving this medication • Do not shake aerosol spray because this affects metered dose | **Sublingual Route** • 1 tablet (0.3-0.4 mg), repeated for total of 3 doses at 5-minute intervals • 1-2 sprays at 5-minute intervals (provides 0.4 mg per dose); maximum 3 sprays within 15 minutes • *Note:* Patients should be instructed to contact EMS if pain is unrelieved or increasing after 1 tablet or sublingual spray |

## Nitroprusside
(Sodium Nitroprusside)

### Indications
- Hypertensive crisis
- To reduce afterload in heart failure and acute pulmonary edema
- To reduce afterload in acute mitral or aortic valve regurgitation

### Precautions
- May cause hypotension and cyanide toxicity
- May reverse hypoxic pulmonary vasoconstriction in patients with pulmonary disease, exacerbating intrapulmonary shunting, resulting in hypoxemia
- Other side effects include headaches, nausea, vomiting, and abdominal cramps
- Contraindicated in patients who have recently taken phosphodiesterase inhibitors for erectile dysfunction (eg, sildenafil)

### IV Administration
- Begin at 0.1 mcg/kg per minute and titrate upward every 3-5 minutes to desired effect (usually up to 5 mcg/kg per minute, but higher doses up to 10 mcg/kg may be needed)
- Use with an infusion pump; use hemodynamic monitoring for optimal safety
- Action occurs within 1-2 minutes
- Light sensitive; cover drug reservoir and tubing with opaque material

| Drug/Therapy | Indications/Precautions | Adult Dosage |
|---|---|---|
| Norepinephrine | **Indications** <br> • Severe cardiogenic shock and hemodynamically significant hypotension (systolic blood pressure <70 mm Hg) with low total peripheral resistance <br> • Agent of last resort for management of ischemic heart disease and shock <br><br> **Precautions** <br> • Increases myocardial oxygen requirements; raises blood pressure and heart rate <br> • May induce arrhythmias; use with caution in patients with acute ischemia; monitor cardiac output <br> • Extravasation causes tissue necrosis <br> • If extravasation occurs, administer phentolamine 5–10 mg in 10–15 mL saline solution; infiltrate into area <br> • Relatively contraindicated in patients with hypovolemia | **IV Administration (Only Route)** <br> • Initial rate: 0.1–0.5 mcg/kg per minute (for 70-kg patient: 7–35 mcg/min); titrate to response <br> • Do not administer in same IV line as alkaline solutions <br> • Poison/drug-induced hypotension may require higher doses to achieve adequate perfusion |

## Oxygen

Delivered from portable tanks or installed, wall-mounted sources through delivery devices

**Indications**

- Any suspected cardiopulmonary emergency
- Complaints of shortness of breath and suspected ischemic pain
- For ACS: May administer to patients until stable; continue if pulmonary congestion, ongoing ischemia, or oxygen saturation <90%
- For patients with suspected stroke and hypoxemia, arterial oxygen desaturation (oxyhemoglobin saturation ≤94%), or unknown oxyhemoglobin saturation; may consider administration to patients who are not hypoxemic
- After ROSC following resuscitation: Use the minimum inspired oxygen concentration to achieve oxyhemoglobin saturation of 92% to 98%

**Precautions**

- Observe closely when using with pulmonary patients known to be dependent on hypoxic respiratory drive (very rare)
- Pulse oximetry may be inaccurate in low cardiac output states, with vasoconstriction, or with exposure to carbon monoxide

| Device | Flow Rate | O₂ (%) |
|---|---|---|
| Nasal cannula | 1-6 L/min | 21-44 |
| Venturi mask | 4-12 L/min | 24-50 |
| Partial rebreathing mask | 6-10 L/min | 35-60 |
| Nonrebreathing oxygen mask with reservoir | 6-15 L/min | 60-100 |
| Bag-mask with reservoir (bag or tail) | 15 L/min | 95-100 |

*Note*: Pulse oximetry provides a useful method of titrating oxygen administration to maintain physiologic oxygen saturation (see Precautions).

| Drug/Therapy | Indications/Precautions | Adult Dosage |
|---|---|---|
| **P2Y$_{12}$ Receptor Blockers** | **Indications**<br>Adjunctive antiplatelet therapy for ACS patients | |
| **Cangrelor** (Kengreal) | **Precautions/Contraindications**<br>• Do not administer to patients with active pathologic bleeding (eg, peptic ulcer); use with caution in patients with risk of bleeding. | **Cangrelor**<br>• During PCI procedure: 30 mcg/kg IV bolus prior to intervention, followed immediately by 4 mcg/kg per minute infusion for at least 2 hours or for the duration of the PCI, whichever is longer |
| **Clopidogrel** (Plavix) | | |
| **Prasugrel** (Effient) | • Prasugrel is contraindicated in patients with a history of TIA or stroke; use with caution in patients ≥75 years old or <60 kg because of uncertain benefit and increased risk of intracranial hemorrhage and fatal bleeding | |
| **Ticagrelor** (Brilinta) | • Use with caution in the presence of hepatic impairment<br>• When CABG is planned, withhold P2Y$_{12}$ receptor blockers for 5 days (for clopidogrel and ticagrelor) or 7 days (for prasugrel) before CABG unless need for revascularization outweighs the risk of excess bleeding | |
| **Cangrelor** | • Adjunct IV antiplatelet agent administered to patients during PCI who have not been previously treated with an oral P2Y$_{12}$ inhibitor<br>• Reversible antiplatelet agent with very short half-life (3-6 minutes) | |

(continued)

## P2Y$_{12}$ Receptor Blockers
*(continued)*

• When transitioning to oral P2Y$_{12}$ inhibitor, clopidogrel and prasugrel must be given immediately *after* discontinuation of cangrelor infusion. Ticagrelor may be administered at any time during cangrelor infusion or immediately after discontinuation of the cangrelor infusion

**Clopidogrel**
• For STEMI or moderate- to high-risk NSTE-ACS, including patients receiving fibrinolysis
• Limited evidence in patients ≥75 years old
• Substitute for aspirin if patient is unable to take aspirin

**Clopidogrel**
• STEMI or moderate- to high-risk NSTE-ACS patients <75 years old: Administer loading dose of 300 to 600 mg orally followed by maintenance dose of 75 mg orally daily; full effects will not develop for several days
• ED patients with suspected ACS unable to take aspirin: loading dose 300 mg

**Prasugrel**
• May be substituted for clopidogrel after angiography in patients with NSTE-ACS or STEMI who are not at high risk for bleeding
• Not recommended for STEMI patients managed with fibrinolysis or for NSTE-ACS patients before angiography
• No data to support use in ED or prehospital setting

**Prasugrel**
• STEMI or NSTE-ACS patients <75 years old managed with PCI: Administer loading dose of 60 mg PO followed by maintenance dose of 10 mg PO daily; full effects will not develop for several days
• Consider dose reduction to 5 mg PO daily in patients weighing <60 kg

*(continued)*

| Drug/Therapy | Indications/Precautions | Adult Dosage |
|---|---|---|
| **P2Y$_{12}$ Receptor Blockers** *(continued)* | Ticagrelor<br>May be administered to patients with NSTE-ACS or STEMI who are treated with early invasive strategy | Ticagrelor<br>• STEMI or NSTE-ACS patients <75 years old: Administer loading dose of 180 mg PO followed by maintenance dose 90 mg PO twice daily<br>• Maintenance dose of aspirin should be <100 mg/day due to drug interaction with higher doses |
| **Prasugrel**<br>(Effient)<br>(see **P2Y$_{12}$ Receptor Blockers**) | | |

## Procainamide

### Indications

- Useful for treatment of a wide variety of arrhythmias, including stable monomorphic VT with normal QT interval and preserved LV function
- May use for treatment of reentry SVT uncontrolled by adenosine and vagal maneuvers if blood pressure stable
- Stable wide-complex tachycardia of unknown origin
- Atrial fibrillation with rapid rate in Wolff-Parkinson-White syndrome

### Precautions

- If cardiac or renal dysfunction is present, reduce maximum total dose to 12 mg/kg and maintenance infusion to 1-2 mg/min
- Proarrhythmic, especially in setting of AMI, hypokalemia, or hypomagnesemia
- May induce hypotension in patients with impaired LV function
- Use with caution with other drugs that prolong QT interval (eg, amiodarone); expert consultation advised

### Recurrent VF/pVT

- 20 mg/min IV infusion (maximum total dose: 17 mg/kg)
- In urgent situations, up to 50 mg/min may be administered to total dose of 17 mg/kg

### Other Indications

- 20 mg/min IV infusion until one of the following occurs:
  - Arrhythmia suppression
  - Hypotension
  - QRS widens by >50%
  - Total dose of 17 mg/kg is given
- Use in cardiac arrest limited by need for slow infusion and uncertain efficacy

### Maintenance Infusion

1-4 mg/min (dilute in $D_5W$ or NS); reduce dose in presence of renal or hepatic insufficiency

---

## Propranolol
(see *β-Blockers*)

---

## Ramipril
(see *ACE Inhibitors*)

| Drug/Therapy | Indications/Precautions | Adult Dosage |
|---|---|---|
| **Reteplase, Recombinant** (Retavase) | *(see Fibrinolytic Agents)* | |
| **Sodium Bicarbonate** | **Indications** <br> • Known preexisting hyperkalemia <br> • Known preexisting bicarbonate-responsive acidosis (eg, diabetic ketoacidosis or overdose of tricyclic antidepressant, aspirin, cocaine, or diphenhydramine) <br> • Prolonged resuscitation with effective ventilation; on return of spontaneous circulation after long arrest interval <br> • Not useful or effective in hypercarbic acidosis (eg, cardiac arrest and CPR without intubation) <br><br> **Precautions** <br> • Adequate ventilation and CPR, not bicarbonate, are the major "buffer agents" in cardiac arrest. <br> • Not recommended for routine use in cardiac arrest patients | **IV Administration** <br> • 1 mEq/kg IV bolus <br> • If rapidly available, use arterial blood gas analysis to guide bicarbonate therapy (calculated base deficits or bicarbonate concentration); during cardiac arrest, ABG results are not reliable indicators of acidosis |

## Sotalol
Seek expert consultation

### Indications
Treatment of supraventricular arrhythmias and ventricular arrhythmias in patients without structural heart disease

### Precautions/Contraindications
- Should be avoided in patients with poor perfusion because of significant negative inotropic effects
- Adverse effects include bradycardia, hypotension, and arrhythmias (torsades de pointes)
- Use with caution with other drugs that prolong QT interval (eg, procainamide, amiodarone)
- May become toxic in patients with renal impairment; contraindicated if creatinine clearance <40 mL/min

### IV Administration
- 1.5 mg/kg over 5 minutes
- Check hospital protocol for infusion rate; package insert recommends slow infusion, but literature supports more rapid infusion of 1.5 mg/kg over 5 minutes or less

## Tenecteplase
(TNKase)
(see *Fibrinolytic Agents*)

## Thrombolytic Agents
(see *Fibrinolytic Agents*)

## Ticagrelor
(Brilinta)
(see *P2Y$_{12}$ Receptor Blockers*)

| Drug/Therapy | Indications/Precautions | Adult Dosage |
|---|---|---|
| **Tirofiban** (Aggrastat) | **Indications** <br> For high-risk NSTE-ACS and patients undergoing PCI <br><br> **Actions/Precautions** <br> Platelet function recovers within 4-8 hours after discontinuation <br><br> **Contraindications** <br> Active internal bleeding or history of bleeding disorder in past 30 days, history of intracranial hemorrhage or other bleeding, surgical procedure or trauma within 1 month, platelet count <150 000/mm³, hypersensitivity and concomitant use of another GP IIb/IIIa inhibitor (also see Acute Coronary Syndromes: Treatment Recommendations) | **Note: Check package insert for current indications, doses, and duration of therapy.** Optimal duration of therapy has not been established. <br> • **PCI:** 25 mcg/kg administered over 3 minutes; then 0.15 mcg/kg per minute IV infusion (for 18-24 hours after PCI) <br> • Reduce rate of infusion by 50% if creatinine clearance <60 mL/min |
| **Vasopressin** | **Indications** <br> May be useful for hemodynamic support in vasodilatory shock (eg, septic shock) <br><br> **Precautions/Contraindications** <br> • Potent peripheral vasoconstrictor; increased peripheral vascular resistance may provoke cardiac ischemia and angina <br> • Not recommended for responsive patients with coronary artery disease | **Vasodilatory shock:** Continuous infusion of 0.02-0.04 units/min <br><br> **IV Administration** |

**Verapamil**

**Indications**

- Alternative drug (after adenosine) to terminate reentry SVT with narrow QRS complex and adequate blood pressure and *preserved LV function*
- May control ventricular response in patients with atrial fibrillation, flutter, or multifocal atrial tachycardia

**Precautions**

- Give *only* to patients with narrow-complex reentry SVT or known supraventricular arrhythmias
- Do not use for wide-QRS tachycardias of uncertain origin, and avoid use for Wolff-Parkinson-White syndrome and atrial fibrillation, sick sinus syndrome, or second- or third-degree AV block without pacemaker
- May decrease myocardial contractility, and can produce peripheral vasodilation and hypotension; IV calcium may restore blood pressure in toxic cases
- Concurrent IV administration with IV β-blockers may produce severe hypotension; use with extreme caution in patients receiving oral β-blockers

**IV Administration**

- **First dose**: 2.5-5 mg IV bolus over 2 minutes (over 3 minutes in older patients)
- **Second dose**: 5-10 mg, if needed, every 15-30 minutes; maximum total dose: 20 mg
- **Alternative**: 5 mg bolus every 15 minutes to total dose of 30 mg

## Useful Calculations and Formulas

| Calculation | Formula | Comments |
|---|---|---|
| Anion gap (serum) concentration in mEq/L | $[Na^+] - ([Cl^-] + [HCO_3^-])$ | Normal range: 10–15 mEq/L. A gap >15 suggests a high anion gap metabolic acidosis. |
| Osmolal gap | $Osmolality_{measured} - Osmolality_{calculated}$<br>Normal = <10 | Osmolal gap normally <10 suggests a high anion gap metabolic acidosis. If osmolal gap is >10, suspect unknown osmotically active substances. |
| Calculated osmolality (in mOsm/L) | $(2 \times [Na^+]) + ([Glucose] \div 18) + (BUN] \div 2.8)$ | Simplified to give effective osmolality; Normal = 272–300 mOsm/L |

(continued)

| Calculation | Formula | Comments |
|---|---|---|
| Determination of *predicted* pH | $(40 - P_{CO_2}) \times 0.008 = \pm \Delta$ in pH from 7.4 | For every 1 mm Hg uncompensated change in $P_{CO_2}$ from 40, pH will change by 0.008.<br><br>Measured pH less than predicted pH: Metabolic acidosis is present.<br><br>Measured pH greater than predicted pH: Metabolic alkalosis is present. |

# ACLS Management of Hyperkalemia

## Emergency Treatments and Treatment Sequence for Hyperkalemia

| Therapy | Dose | Effect Mechanism | Onset of Effect | Duration of Effect |
|---------|------|-----------------|-----------------|--------------------|
| Calcium | • Calcium chloride (10%): 5-10 mL IV<br>• Calcium gluconate (10%): 15-30 mL IV | Antagonism of toxic effects of hyperkalemia at cell membrane | 1-3 min | 30-60 min |
| Sodium bicarbonate | • Begin with 50 mEq IV<br>• May repeat in 15 minutes | Redistribution: intracellular shift | 5-10 min | 1-2 h |
| Insulin plus glucose (use 2 units insulin per 5 g glucose) | 10 units regular insulin IV plus 25 g dextrose (50 mL D$_{50}$) | Redistribution: intracellular shift | 30 min | 4-6 h |
| Nebulized albuterol | • 10-20 mg over 15 min<br>• May repeat | Redistribution: intracellular shift | 15 min | 15-90 min |

(continued)

| Therapy | Dose | Effect Mechanism | Onset of Effect | Duration of Effect |
|---|---|---|---|---|
| Diuresis with furosemide | 40-80 mg IV bolus | Removal from body | At start of diuresis | Until end of diuresis |
| Cation-exchange resin (Kayexalate) | 15-50 g PO or PR plus sorbitol | Removal from body | 1-2 h | 4-6 h |
| Peritoneal or hemodialysis | Per institutional protocol | Removal from body | At start of dialysis | Until end of dialysis |

# Common Toxidromes*

*Whenever possible, contact a medical toxicologist or poison center (eg, in USA: 1-800-222-1222) for advice when treating suspected severe poisoning.*

## Cardiac Signs

| Tachycardia and/or Hypertension | Bradycardia and/or Hypotension | Cardiac Conduction Delays (Wide QRS) |
| --- | --- | --- |
| • Amphetamines<br>• Anticholinergic drugs<br>• Antihistamines<br>• Cocaine<br>• Theophylline/caffeine<br>• Withdrawal states | • β-Blockers<br>• Calcium channel blockers<br>• Clonidine<br>• Digoxin and related glycosides<br>• Organophosphates and carbamates | • Cocaine<br>• Cyclic antidepressants<br>• Local anesthetics<br>• Propoxyphene<br>• Vaughan-Williams Class Ia and Ic agents (eg, quinidine, flecainide) |

## Central Nervous System/Metabolic Signs

| Seizures | Central Nervous System and/or Respiratory Depression | Metabolic Acidosis |
| --- | --- | --- |
| • Cyclic antidepressants<br>• Isoniazid<br>• Selective and nonselective norepinephrine reuptake inhibitors (eg, bupropion)<br>• Withdrawal states | • Antidepressants (several classes)<br>• Benzodiazepines<br>• Carbon monoxide<br>• Ethanol<br>• Methanol<br>• Opioids<br>• Oral hypoglycemics | • Cyanide<br>• Ethylene glycol<br>• Iron<br>• Metformin<br>• Methanol<br>• Salicylates |

*Whenever possible, consult a medical toxicologist or call poison center (eg, in USA: 1-800-222-1222) for advice before administering antidotes.*

| Antidote | Common Indications: Toxicity due to | Adult Dose* | Pediatric Dose* Do not exceed adult dose | Notes |
|---|---|---|---|---|
| **Atropine** | • β-Blockers<br>• Calcium channel blockers<br>• Clonidine<br>• Digoxin | 1 mg IV every 3-5 minutes with a maximum of 3 mg | 0.02 mg/kg IV (minimum dose 0.1 mg) every 2-3 minutes | Use for hemodynamically significant bradycardia. Higher doses often required for organophosphate or carbamate poisoning. |
| **Calcium** | • β-Blockers<br>• Calcium channel blockers | • Calcium chloride (10%): 1-2 g (10-20 mL) IV<br>• Calcium gluconate (10%): 3-6 g (30-60 mL) IV<br>• Follow initial dose with same dose by continuous hourly infusion | • Calcium chloride (10%): 20 mg/kg (0.2 mL/kg) IV<br>• Calcium gluconate (10%): 60 mg/kg (0.6 mL/kg) IV<br>• Follow initial dose with same dose by continuous hourly infusion | Use for hypotension. Avoid calcium chloride when possible if using peripheral IV, particularly in children. Higher doses may be required for calcium channel blocker overdose (use caution and monitor serum calcium). |

*(continued)*

# Rapid Dosing Guide for Antidotes Used in Emergency Cardiovascular Care for Treatment of Toxic Ingestions (continued)

(continued)

| Antidote | Common Indications: Toxicity due to | Adult Dose* | Pediatric Dose* Do not exceed adult dose | Notes |
|---|---|---|---|---|
| Digoxin Immune Fab | • Digoxin and related glycosides | **If amount of digoxin ingested is known:** <br> • **If amount of digoxin ingested is unknown or if chronic intoxication with a known digoxin level:** <br> Dose (vials, administered IV) = $$\frac{\text{(serum digoxin concentration [ng/mL]} \times \text{weight [kg])}}{100}$$ • **Unknown dose and level, cardiovascular collapse:** 10-20 vials IV | • **If amount of digoxin ingested is known:** <br> Give 1 vial IV for every 0.5 mg digoxin ingested. | |
| Flumazenil | • Benzodiazepines | 0.2 mg IV every 15 seconds, up to 3 mg total dose | 0.01 mg/kg IV every 15 seconds, up to 0.05 mg/kg total dose | Do not use for unknown overdose, suspected TCA overdose, or patients who are benzodiazepine dependent because of risk of precipitating seizures. |
| Glucagon | • β-Blockers <br> • Calcium channel blockers | 3-10 mg IV bolus, followed by 3-5 mg per hour IV infusion | 0.05-0.15 mg/kg IV bolus, followed by 0.05-0.1 mg/kg per hour IV infusion | Bolus often causes vomiting. |

| Hydroxo-cobalamin | • Cyanide | 5 g IV | 70 mg/kg IV | Dilute in 100 mL normal saline; infuse over 15 minutes. Toxicologist or other specialist may follow with sodium thiosulfate (separate IV). |
|---|---|---|---|---|
| **Lipid Emulsion** | • Local anesthetics<br>• Possibly other toxicants if failing standard resuscitation | 1.5 mL/kg lean body mass of 20% emulsion of long-chain triglycerides IV bolus over 1 minute followed by infusion of 0.25 mL/kg per minute for 30-60 minutes. The bolus can be repeated once or twice as needed for persistent cardiovascular collapse; suggested maximum total dose is 10 mL/kg over first hour. | | |
| **Insulin** | • β-Blockers<br>• Calcium channel blockers | 1 unit/kg IV bolus, then 0.5-1 units/kg per hour IV infusion, titrated to blood pressure | | Give dextrose 0.5 g/kg with insulin. Start dextrose infusion 0.5 g/kg per hour and check blood sugar frequently. Replace potassium to maintain serum potassium 2.5-2.8 mEq/L. |

*(continued)*

| Antidote | Common Indications: Toxicity due to | Adult Dose* | Pediatric Dose* Do not exceed adult dose | Notes |
|---|---|---|---|---|
| **Naloxone** | • Opioids | • IM or IV: 0.04-0.4 mg, repeated every 2-3 minutes if necessary • Intranasal: 2 mg, repeated every 3-5 minutes if necessary | 0.1 mg/kg IV (up to 2 mg per dose). Repeat every 2-3 minutes. For partial reversal of respiratory depression (eg, procedural sedation), 0.001-0.005 mg/kg (1-5 mcg/kg) IV. Titrate to effect. | Use only for respiratory depression or loss of airway reflexes. May also be given by IO, nebulized, or endotracheal routes. |
| **Sodium Bicarbonate** | • Cyclic anti-depressants | 1 mEq/kg IV (1 mL/kg of 8.4% solution); consider infusion following initial dose | | Repeat as needed until QRS narrows. Avoid sodium > 155 mEq/L or pH > 7.55. Dilute before administration in small children. |

*(continued)*

| | | | | |
|---|---|---|---|---|
| **Sodium Nitrite** | • Cyanide | 300 mg IV over 3-5 minutes (10 mL of 3% solution) | 10 mg/kg (0.33 mL/kg of 10% solution) IV over 3-5 minutes | Hydroxocobalamin preferred to sodium nitrite, if available. May give inhaled amyl nitrite as temporizing measure while establishing vascular access. Follow with sodium thiosulfate administration. Reduced dose required for children with anemia. |
| **Sodium Thiosulfate** | • Cyanide | 12.5 g (50 mL of 25% solution) IV over 10 minutes | 400 mg/kg (1.65 mL/kg of 25% solution) IV over 10 minutes | Use separate IV from hydroxocobalamin. Consider expert consultation. |

*These doses are often different from doses used in other emergency cardiovascular care situations. The ideal dose has not been determined for many indications; the doses above may not be ideal. Most antidotes may be repeated as needed to achieve and maintain the desired clinical effect. Unless otherwise noted, IV doses may also be given via the IO route. Contact medical toxicologist, call poison center (eg, in USA: 1-800-222-1222), or refer to written treatment guidance for specific dosing advice.

## Pre-event Equipment Checklist for Endotracheal Intubation

- ☐ Universal precautions (gloves, mask, eye protection)
- ☐ Cardiac monitor, pulse oximeter, and blood pressure monitoring device
- ☐ Continuous waveform capnography device or, if not available, exhaled $CO_2$ detector (qualitative) or esophageal detector device (aspiration technique)
- ☐ Intravenous and intraosseous infusion equipment
- ☐ Oxygen supply, bag mask (appropriate size)
- ☐ Oral/tracheal suction equipment (appropriate size); confirm that it is working
- ☐ Oral and nasopharyngeal airways (appropriate size)
- ☐ Endotracheal tubes with stylets (all sizes) 0.5 mm (i.d.) above and below anticipated size for patient
- ☐ Laryngoscope (curved and straight blades) and/or video laryngoscope; backup laryngoscope available
- ☐ 10-mL syringes to test inflate endotracheal tube balloon
- ☐ Adhesive/cloth tape or commercial tube holder to secure tube
- ☐ Towels, sheets, or pad to align by placing under head or torso
- ☐ Rescue equipment as needed for difficult airway management or anticipated complications (eg, supraglottic airway, transtracheal ventilation, and/or cricothyrotomy equipment)

## Rapid Sequence Intubation Protocol

| Pre-event preparation | 1. | Obtain brief medical history and perform focused physical examination. |
|---|---|---|
| | 2. | Prepare equipment, monitors, personnel, medications. |
| | 3. | If neck injury not suspected: place in sniffing position. |
| | | If neck injury suspected: stabilize cervical spine. |
| Preoxygenate | 4. | Preoxygenate with $FiO_2$ of 100% by mask (nonrebreather preferred). If ventilatory assistance is necessary, ventilate gently. |
| Premedicate | 5. | Premedicate with atropine or glycopyrrolate as appropriate; wait briefly to allow adequate drug effect after administration. |
| Pharmacologic sedation/anesthesia/neuromuscular blockade and protection/positioning | 6. | Administer sedation/anesthesia by IV push. |
| | 7. | Give neuromuscular blocking agent by IV push. |
| | 8. | Assess for apnea, jaw relaxation, and absence of movement (patient sufficiently relaxed to proceed with intubation). |
| Placement of endotracheal tube | 9. | Perform endotracheal intubation. If during intubation oxygen saturation is inadequate, stop laryngoscopy and start ventilation with bag-mask. Monitor pulse oximetry and ensure adequate oxygen saturation. Reattempt intubation. Once intubated, inflate cuff to minimal occlusive volume. |
| | | Be prepared to place rescue airway if intubation attempts are unsuccessful. |
| Placement confirmation | 10. | Confirm placement of endotracheal tube by |
| | | • Direct visualization of endotracheal tube passing through vocal cords |
| | | • Chest rise/fall with each ventilation (bilateral) |
| | | • 5-point auscultation: anterior chest L and R, midaxillary line L and R, and over the epigastrium (no breath sounds over epigastrium); look for tube condensation |
| | | • Using end-tidal $CO_2$ measured by quantitative continuous waveform capnography; if waveform capnography not available, use qualitative exhaled $CO_2$ detector or esophageal detector device (aspiration technique) |
| | | • Monitoring $O_2$ saturation (indirect evidence of adequate oxygenation) |
| Postintubation management | 11. | Prevent dislodgement: |
| | | • Secure endotracheal tube with adhesive/cloth tape or commercial endotracheal tube holder |
| | | • Continue cervical spine immobilization |
| | | • Continue sedation; add paralytics if necessary |
| | | • Check cuff inflation pressure |

## Pharmacologic Agents Used for Rapid Sequence Intubation

| Drug | IV/IO Push* | Onset | Duration | Side Effects | Comments |
|------|-------------|-------|----------|--------------|----------|
| **Premedication Agents** | | | | | |
| Atropine | 0.01-0.02 mg/kg (minimum: 0.1 mg; maximum single dose: 0.5 mg) | 1-2 min | 2-4 hours | Paradoxical bradycardia can occur with doses <0.1 mg Tachycardia, agitation | Antisialogogue Inhibits bradycardic response to hypoxia, laryngoscopy, and succinylcholine May cause pupil dilation |
| Glycopyrrolate | 0.005-0.01 mg/kg (maximum: 0.2 mg) | 1-2 min | 4-6 hours | Tachycardia | Antisialogogue Inhibits bradycardic response to hypoxia, laryngoscopy, and succinylcholine |
| Lidocaine | 1-2 mg/kg (maximum: 100 mg) | 1-2 min | 10-20 min | Myocardial and CNS depression Seizures with high doses | May decrease ICP during RSI May decrease pain on propofol injection |

(continued)

| Drug | IV/IO Push* | Onset | Duration | Side Effects | Comments |
|---|---|---|---|---|---|
| **Sedative/Anesthetic Agents** | | | | | |
| **Etomidate** | 0.2-0.4 mg/kg Caution: Limit to 1 dose | <1 min | 5-10 min | Myoclonic activity Inhibition of cortisol synthesis for up to 12 hours | Ultrashort acting No analgesic properties Decreases cerebral metabolic rate and ICP Generally maintains hemodynamic stability |
| **Fentanyl citrate** | 2-5 mcg/kg | 1-3 min | 30-60 min | Chest wall rigidity possible with high-dose rapid infusions | Minimum histamine release May lower blood pressure (especially with higher doses or in conjunction with midazolam) |
| **Ketamine** | 1-2 mg/kg | 30-60 sec | 10-20 min | Hypertension, tachycardia Increased secretions and laryngospasm Emergence reactions and hallucinations | Dissociative anesthetic agent Limited respiratory depression Bronchodilator May cause myocardial depression in catecholamine-depleted patients Use with caution in patients with potential or increased ICP |

*(continued)*

| Drug | IV/IO Push* | Onset | Duration | Side Effects | Comments |
|------|-------------|-------|----------|--------------|----------|
| Sedative/Anesthetic Agents | | | | | |
| Midazolam | 0.1–0.3 mg/kg (maximum single dose: 10 mg) | 2–5 min | 15–30 min | Hypotension | Hypotension exacerbated in combination with narcotics and barbiturates<br>No analgesic properties<br>Excellent amnesia |
| Propofol | 1–2 mg/kg | <1 min | 5–10 min | Hypotension, especially in patients with inadequate intravascular volume<br>Pain on infusion | No analgesic properties<br>Very short duration of action<br>Less airway reactivity than barbiturates<br>Decreases cerebral metabolic rate and ICP<br>Lidocaine may decrease infusion pain<br>Not recommended in patients with egg/soy allergy |

(continued)

| Drug | IV/IO Push* | Onset | Duration | Side Effects | Comments |
|------|-------------|-------|----------|--------------|----------|
| **Neuromuscular Blocking Agents** | | | | | |
| **Succinylcho-line** | 1-1.5 mg/kg | 45-60 sec | 5-10 min | Muscle fasciculations May cause rhabdomyolysis; rise in intracranial, intraocular, intragastric pressure; life-threatening hyperkalemia | Depolarizing muscle relaxant Rapid onset, short duration of action Avoid in burns, crush injuries after 48 hours, muscular dystrophy and other neuromuscular diseases, hyperkalemia, or family history of malignant hyperthermia Use with caution in renal failure; monitor serum potassium Do not use to maintain paralysis |
| **Vecuronium** | 0.1-0.2 mg/kg | 1-3 min | 45-90 min | Minimal cardiovascular side effects | Nondepolarizing agent The higher the dose, the quicker the onset of action and the longer the duration |
| **Cisatracurium** | 0.4 mg/kg | 2-3 min | 90-120 min | Minimal cardiovascular side effects | Nondepolarizing agent Degrades spontaneously, independent of organ elimination |
| **Rocuronium** | 0.6-1.2 mg/kg | 60-90 sec | 45-120 min | Minimal cardiovascular side effects | Nondepolarizing agent Rapid onset of action |

Abbreviations: CNS, central nervous system; ICP, intracranial pressure; IO, intraosseous; IV, intravenous; RSI, rapid sequence intubation.
*Doses provided are guidelines only. Actual dosing may vary depending on patient's clinical status.

## Capnography to Confirm Endotracheal Tube Placement

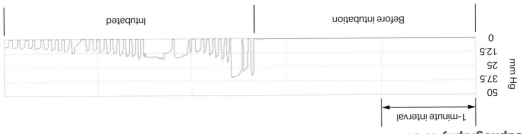

This capnography tracing displays the partial pressure of exhaled carbon dioxide (PETCO$_2$) in mm Hg on the vertical axis over time when intubation is performed. Once the patient is intubated, exhaled carbon dioxide is detected, confirming tracheal tube placement. The PETCO$_2$ varies during the respiratory cycle, with highest values at end-expiration.

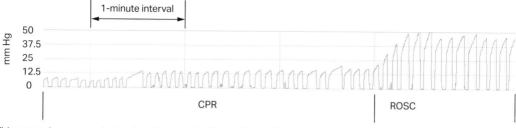

This second capnography tracing displays the PETCO$_2$ in mm Hg on the vertical axis over time. This patient is intubated and receiving CPR. Note that the ventilation rate is approximately 8 to 10 breaths/min. Chest compressions are given continuously at a rate of slightly faster than 100/min but are not visible with this tracing. The initial PETCO$_2$ is less than 12.5 mm Hg during the first minute, indicating very low blood flow. The PETCO$_2$ increases to between 12.5 and 25 mm Hg during the second and third minutes, consistent with the increase in blood flow with ongoing resuscitation. Return of spontaneous circulation (ROSC) occurs during the fourth minute. ROSC is recognized by the abrupt increase in the PETCO$_2$ (visible just after the fourth vertical line) to over 40 mm Hg, which is consistent with a substantial improvement in blood flow.

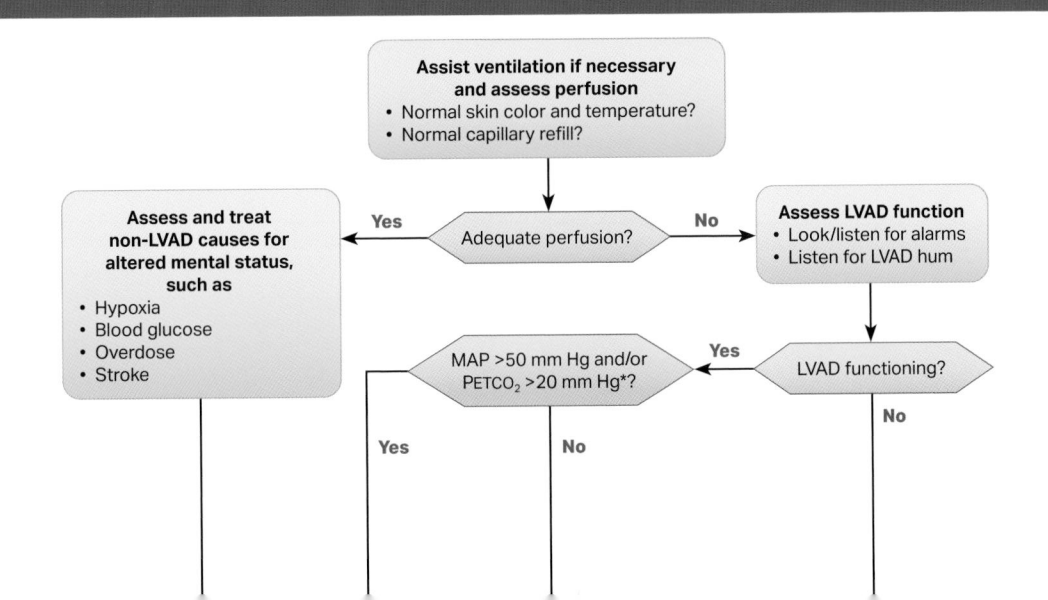

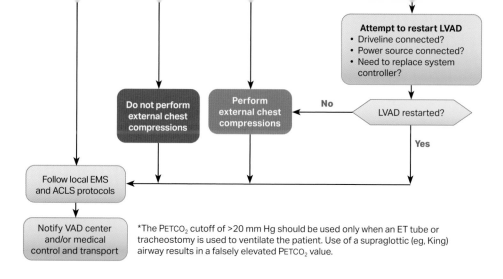

| | | | **Attempt to restart LVAD** |
|---|---|---|---|

**Attempt to restart LVAD**
- Driveline connected?
- Power source connected?
- Need to replace system controller?

**Do not perform external chest compressions**

**Perform external chest compressions**

LVAD restarted?

No

Yes

Follow local EMS and ACLS protocols

Notify VAD center and/or medical control and transport

\*The PETCO₂ cutoff of >20 mm Hg should be used only when an ET tube or tracheostomy is used to ventilate the patient. Use of a supraglottic (eg, King) airway results in a falsely elevated PETCO₂ value.

Abbreviations: ACLS, advanced cardiovascular life support; EMS, emergency medical services; ET, endotracheal; LVAD, left ventricular assist device; VAD, ventricular assist device.

# Neuroprognostication Diagram

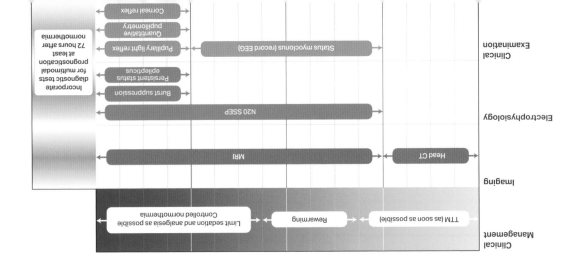

**Clinical Examination**
- Corneal reflex
- Quantitative pupillometry
- Pupillary light reflex
- Status myoclonus (record EEG)

**Electrophysiology**
- Burst suppression
- Persistent status epilepticus
- N20 SSEP

**Imaging**
- MRI
- Head CT

**Clinical Management**
- TTM (as soon as possible)
- Rewarming
- Limit sedation and analgesia as possible
- Controlled normothermia

Incorporate diagnostic tests for multimodal prognostication at least 72 hours after normothermia

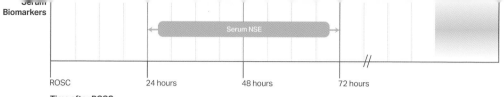

ROSC   24 hours   48 hours   72 hours

**Time after ROSC**

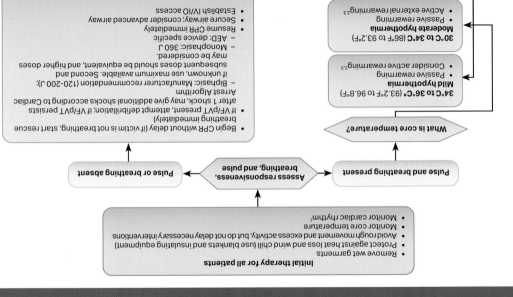

**Initial therapy for all patients**

- Remove wet garments
- Protect against heat loss and wind chill (use blankets and insulating equipment)
- Avoid rough movement and excess activity, but do not delay necessary interventions
- Monitor core temperature
- Monitor cardiac rhythm[1]

**Assess responsiveness, breathing, and pulse**

→ **Pulse or breathing absent**

**Pulse and breathing present**

**Pulse or breathing absent**

- Begin CPR without delay (if victim is not breathing, start rescue breathing immediately)
- If VF/pVT present, attempt defibrillation; if VF/pVT persists after 1 shock, may give additional shocks according to Cardiac Arrest Algorithm
  - Biphasic: Manufacturer recommendation (120-200 J); if unknown, use maximum available. Second and subsequent doses should be equivalent, and higher doses may be considered.
  - Monophasic: 360 J
  - AED: device specific
- Resume CPR immediately
- Secure airway; consider advanced airway
- Establish IV/IO access

**Pulse and breathing present**

**What is core temperature?**

**34°C to 36°C\*** (93.2°F to 96.8°F)
**Mild hypothermia**
- Passive rewarming
- Consider active rewarming[2,3]

**30°C to 34°C** (86°F to 93.2°F)
**Moderate hypothermia**
- Passive rewarming
- Active external rewarming[2,3]

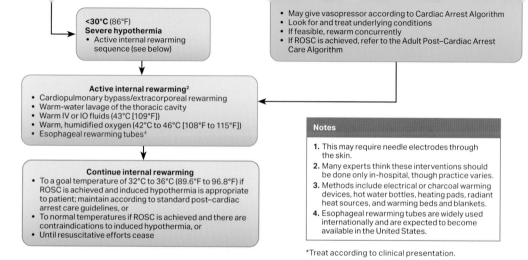

**<30°C (86°F)**
**Severe hypothermia**
- Active internal rewarming sequence (see below)

- May give vasopressor according to Cardiac Arrest Algorithm
- Look for and treat underlying conditions
- If feasible, rewarm concurrently
- If ROSC is achieved, refer to the Adult Post–Cardiac Arrest Care Algorithm

**Active internal rewarming[2]**
- Cardiopulmonary bypass/extracorporeal rewarming
- Warm-water lavage of the thoracic cavity
- Warm IV or IO fluids (43°C [109°F])
- Warm, humidified oxygen (42°C to 46°C [108°F to 115°F])
- Esophageal rewarming tubes[4]

**Continue internal rewarming**
- To a goal temperature of 32°C to 36°C (89.6°F to 96.8°F) if ROSC is achieved and induced hypothermia is appropriate to patient; maintain according to standard post–cardiac arrest care guidelines, or
- To normal temperatures if ROSC is achieved and there are contraindications to induced hypothermia, or
- Until resuscitative efforts cease

#### Notes

1. This may require needle electrodes through the skin.
2. Many experts think these interventions should be done only in-hospital, though practice varies.
3. Methods include electrical or charcoal warming devices, hot water bottles, heating pads, radiant heat sources, and warming beds and blankets.
4. Esophageal rewarming tubes are widely used internationally and are expected to become available in the United States.

*Treat according to clinical presentation.

Abbreviations: AED, automated external defibrillator; CPR, cardiopulmonary resuscitation; IO, intraosseous; IV, intravenous; pVT, pulseless ventricular tachycardia; ROSC, return of spontaneous circulation; VF, ventricular fibrillation.

Ideally, newborn resuscitation takes place in the delivery room or the neonatal intensive care unit, with trained personnel and appropriate equipment readily available. This form of resuscitation is taught in the Neonatal Resuscitation Program (NRP) offered by the American Academy of Pediatrics and the AHA. These pages provide information about initial assessment of the newborn and initial stabilization priorities. Ensuring adequate ventilation of the baby's lungs is the most important and effective action in neonatal resuscitation.

## Initial Assessment and Stabilization

**Airway** (position and clear if required)
**Breathing** (stimulate to breathe)
**Circulation** (assess heart rate and color)

*ABCs of resuscitation*

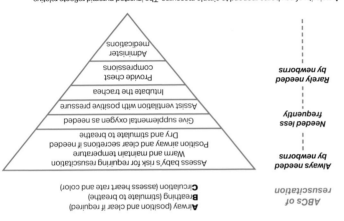

Assess baby's risk for requiring resuscitation
Warm and maintain temperature
Position airway and clear secretions if needed
Dry and stimulate to breathe

Give supplemental oxygen as needed
Assist ventilation with positive pressure
Intubate the trachea
Provide chest compressions
Administer medications

*Always needed by newborns*

*Needed less frequently*

*Rarely needed by newborns*

A majority of newborns respond to simple measures. The inverted pyramid reflects relative frequencies of resuscitative efforts for a newborn.

## Target Preductal SpO$_2$ After Birth

- 1 min    60% to 65%
- 2 min    65% to 70%
- 3 min    70% to 75%
- 4 min    75% to 80%
- 5 min    80% to 85%
- 10 min   85% to 95%

The ranges shown are approximations of the interquartile values reported by Mariani et al and are adjusted to provide easily remembered targets. Mariani G, Dik PB, Ezquer A, et al. Pre-ductal and post-ductal O$_2$ saturation in healthy term neonates after birth. *J Pediatr*. 2007;150(4):418-421.

## Apgar Score

| Sign | 0 | 1 | 2 |
|------|---|---|---|
| Color | Blue or pale | Acrocyanotic | Completely pink |
| Heart rate | Absent | <100/min | >100/min |
| Reflex irritability | No response | Grimace | Cry or active withdrawal |
| Muscle tone | Limp | Some flexion | Active motion |
| Respiration | Absent | Weak cry; hypoventilation | Good, crying |

From Lesson 1: overview and principles of resuscitation. *Textbook of Neonatal Resuscitation*. In: Kattwinkel J, ed. 6th ed. American Academy of Pediatrics and American Heart Association; 2011:35.

Note on assessing color: Evaluating the color of a newly born infant, especially one who is transitioning after birth, is difficult and often subjective. One method is to look for pink color around the mouth, palms, and soles.

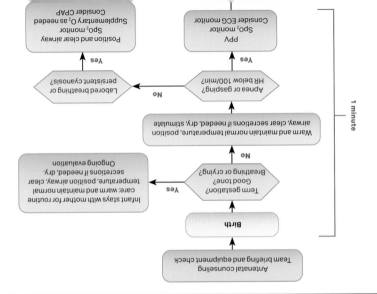

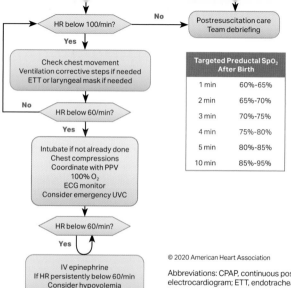

| Targeted Preductal SpO$_2$ After Birth | |
|---|---|
| 1 min | 60%-65% |
| 2 min | 65%-70% |
| 3 min | 70%-75% |
| 4 min | 75%-80% |
| 5 min | 80%-85% |
| 10 min | 85%-95% |

© 2020 American Heart Association

Abbreviations: CPAP, continuous positive airway pressure; ECG, electrocardiogram; ETT, endotracheal tube; HR, heart rate; IV, intravenous; PPV, positive-pressure ventilation; UVC, umbilical vein catheter.

## Initial CPR

**Ventilation rate:** 40 to 60/min when performed without compressions

**Compression rate:** 120 events/min (90 compressions interspersed with 30 ventilations)

**Compression-to-ventilation ratio:** 3:1 (pause compressions for ventilation)

**Medications (epinephrine, volume):** Indicated if heart rate remains less than 60/min despite adequate ventilation with 100% oxygen and chest compressions

## Estimation of Proper Endotracheal Tube Size and Depth of Insertion Based on Infant's Gestational Age and Weight

| Gestational Age (wk) | ETT Insertion Depth at Lips (cm) | Infant's Weight (g) |
|---|---|---|
| 23-24 | 5.5 | 500-600 |
| 25-26 | 6.0 | 700-800 |
| 27-29 | 6.5 | 900-1000 |
| 30-32 | 7.0 | 1100-1400 |
| 33-34 | 7.5 | 1500-1800 |
| 35-37 | 8.0 | 1900-2400 |
| 38-40 | 8.5 | 2500-3100 |
| 41-43 | 9.0 | 3200-4200 |

Initial ETT insertion depth ("tip to lip") for orotracheal intubation. Abbreviation: ETT, endotracheal tube.

Adapted from Kempley ST, Moreiras JW, Petrone FL. Endotracheal tube length for neonatal intubation. *Resuscitation* 2008;77(3):369-373. With permission from Elsevier.

## Endotracheal Tube Size for Infants of Various Weights and Gestational Ages

| Weight (g) | Gestational Age (wk) | ETT Size (mm) (internal diameter) |
|---|---|---|
| <1000 | >28 | 2.5 |
| 1000-2000 | 28-34 | 3.0 |
| >2000 | >34 | 3.5 |

Abbreviation: ETT, endotracheal tube.

## Medications Used During or After Resuscitation of the Newborn

| Medications | Dose/Route* | Concentration | Weight (kg) | Total IV/IO Volume (mL) | Precautions |
|---|---|---|---|---|---|
| **Epinephrine** | IV/IO (UVC preferred route) 0.01-0.03 mg/kg<br>Higher IV/IO doses not recommended<br>Endotracheal 0.05-0.1 mg/kg | 0.1 mg/mL | 1<br>2<br>3<br>4 | 0.1-0.3<br>0.2-0.6<br>0.3-0.9<br>0.4-1.2 | • Give rapidly<br>• Repeat every 3-5 minutes if HR <60 with compressions |
| **Volume expanders**<br>Isotonic crystalloid (normal saline) or blood | 10-20 mL/kg IV/IO | | 1<br>2<br>3<br>4 | 10<br>20<br>30<br>40 | • Indicated for shock<br>• Give over 5-10 minutes<br>• Reassess after each bolus<br>• Use an initial dose of 10 mL/kg<br>• If there are no improvements, an additional 10 mL/kg may be administered |
| **Special considerations after restoring vital signs** | | | | | |
| **Dextrose**<br>(10% solution) | 0.2 g/kg, followed by 5 mL/kg per hour D$_{10}$ IV/IO infusion | 0.1 g/mL | 1<br>2<br>3<br>4 | 2<br>4<br>6<br>8 | • Indicated for blood glucose <40 mg/dL<br>• Check blood glucose 20 minutes after bolus |

Abbreviations: HR, heart rate; IO, intraosseous; IV, intravenous; UVC, umbilical vein catheter.

*Endotracheal dose may not result in effective plasma concentration of drug, so vascular access should be established as soon as possible. Drugs given endotracheally require higher dosing than when given IV/IO.

Use this algorithm to determine the likelihood of congenital heart disease in the cyanotic neonate.

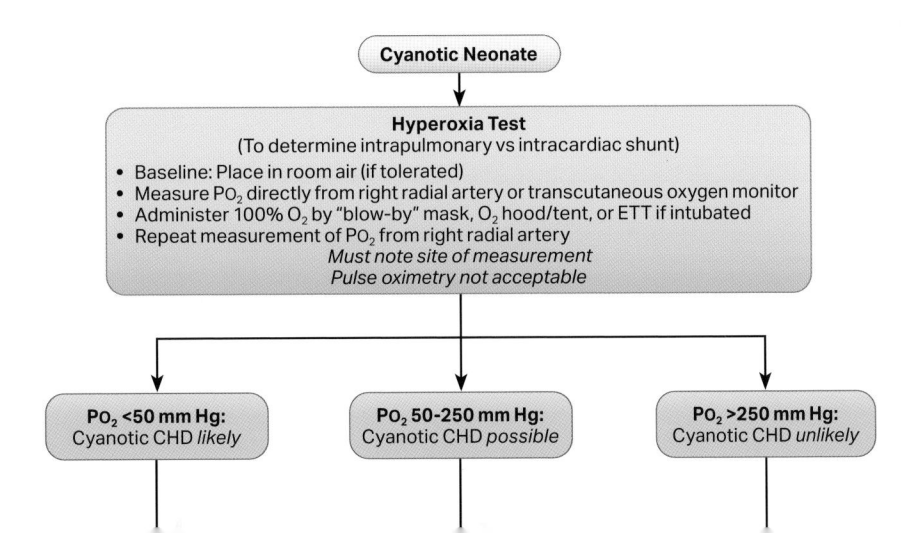

**Cyanotic Neonate**

**Hyperoxia Test**
(To determine intrapulmonary vs intracardiac shunt)
- Baseline: Place in room air (if tolerated)
- Measure $PO_2$ directly from right radial artery or transcutaneous oxygen monitor
- Administer 100% $O_2$ by "blow-by" mask, $O_2$ hood/tent, or ETT if intubated
- Repeat measurement of $PO_2$ from right radial artery
  *Must note site of measurement*
  *Pulse oximetry not acceptable*

$PO_2$ <50 mm Hg:
Cyanotic CHD *likely*

$PO_2$ 50-250 mm Hg:
Cyanotic CHD *possible*

$PO_2$ >250 mm Hg:
Cyanotic CHD *unlikely*

| | Obtain expert consultation | Obtain expert consultation | Titrate oxygen therapy to |
| | Give prostaglandin E₁ (PGE₁) | Consider PGE₁ administration | avoid hypoxia or hyperoxia |
| | | | Avoid hypercarbia |

- Obtain expert consultation
- Give prostaglandin E₁ (PGE₁)

- Obtain expert consultation
- Consider PGE₁ administration

- Titrate oxygen therapy to avoid hypoxia or hyperoxia
- Avoid hypercarbia

Abbreviation: CHD, congenital heart disease; ETT, endotracheal tube.

## Comparison of Differential and Reverse Differential Cyanosis

(10% or greater oxygen saturation difference between right arm vs right or left leg)

| | Preductal Saturation (eg, right arm) | Postductal Saturation (eg, right or left leg) | Differential Diagnosis | Initial Treatment |
|---|---|---|---|---|
| **Differential Cyanosis** | Higher | Lower | • Left-sided obstructive lesion (eg, coarctation of the aorta, interrupted aortic arch, critical aortic stenosis, hypoplastic left heart syndrome) with patent ductus arteriosus<br>• Persistent pulmonary hypertension of the newborn with patent ductus arteriosus | • Administer prostaglandin E₁<br>• Obtain expert consultation |
| **Reverse Differential Cyanosis** | Lower | Higher | • Transposition of the great arteries with left-sided obstructive lesion and patent ductus arteriosus<br>• Transposition of the great arteries with persistent pulmonary hypertension of the newborn and patent ductus arteriosus | |

## Initial Assessment

Primary cardiac arrest in children is much less common than in adults. Cardiac arrest in infants and children does not usually result from a primary cardiac cause; rather, it is the end result of progressive respiratory failure or shock. To prevent pediatric cardiac arrest, providers must detect and treat respiratory failure, respiratory arrest, and shock in a timely manner.

### Conditions Indicating Need for Rapid Assessment and Potential Cardiopulmonary Support

- Irregular respirations or rate greater than 60 breaths/min
- Heart rate ranges (particularly if associated with poor perfusion)
  - Child 2 years or younger: less than 80/min or greater than 180/min
  - Child older than 2 years: less than 60/min or greater than 160/min
- Poor perfusion, with weak or absent distal pulses
- Increased work of breathing (retractions, nasal flaring, grunting)
- Abnormal respirations (eg, bradypnea, seesaw breathing)
- Cyanosis or a decrease in oxyhemoglobin saturation
- Altered level of consciousness (unusual irritability or lethargy or failure to respond to parents or painful procedures)
- Seizures
- Fever with petechiae
- Trauma
- Burns involving more than 10% of body surface area

### Normal Heart Rates*

| Age | Awake Rate (beats/min) | Sleeping Rate (beats/min) |
|---|---|---|
| Neonate | 100-205 | 90-160 |
| Infant | 100-180 | 90-160 |
| Toddler | 98-140 | 80-120 |
| Preschooler | 80-120 | 65-100 |
| School-age child | 75-118 | 58-90 |
| Adolescent | 60-100 | 50-90 |

*Always consider the patient's normal range and clinical condition. Heart rate will normally increase with fever or stress.

### Normal Respiratory Rates*

| Age | Rate (breaths/min) |
|---|---|
| Infant | 30-53 |
| Toddler | 22-37 |
| Preschooler | 20-28 |
| School-age child | 18-25 |
| Adolescent | 12-20 |

*Consider the patient's normal range. The child's respiratory rate is expected to increase in the presence of fever or stress.
Data from Fleming S et al. Lancet. 2011;377(9770):1011-1018.

### Normal Blood Pressures

| Age | Systolic Pressure (mm Hg)* | Diastolic Pressure (mm Hg)* | Mean Arterial Pressure (mm Hg)† |
|---|---|---|---|
| Birth (12 h, <1000 g) | 39-59 | 16-36 | 28-42‡ |
| Birth (12 h, 3 kg) | 60-76 | 31-45 | 48-57 |
| Neonate (96 h) | 67-84 | 35-53 | 45-60 |
| Infant (1-12 mo) | 72-104 | 37-56 | 50-62 |
| Toddler (1-2 y) | 86-106 | 42-63 | 49-62 |
| Preschooler (3-5 y) | 89-112 | 46-72 | 58-69 |
| School-age child (6-9 y) | 97-115 | 57-76 | 66-72 |
| Preadolescent (10-12 y) | 102-120 | 61-80 | 71-79 |
| Adolescent (12-15 y) | 110-131 | 64-83 | 73-84 |

These 3 tables are from Hazinski MF. Children are different. In: Nursing Care of the Critically Ill Child. 3rd ed. Mosby; 2013:1-18, copyright Elsevier.

*Systolic and diastolic blood pressure ranges assume 50th percentile for height for children 1 year and older.

†Mean arterial pressures (diastolic pressure + [difference between systolic and diastolic pressures ÷ 3]) for 1 year and older, assuming 50th percentile for height.

‡Approximately equal to postconception age in weeks (may add 5 mm Hg).

Data from Gemelli M et al. Eur J Pediatr. 1990;149(5)318-320; Versmold HT et al. Pediatrics. 1981;67(5):607-613; Haque IU, Zaritsky AL. Pediatr Crit Care Med. 2007;8(2):138-144; and National Heart, Lung, and Blood Institute: The Fourth Report on the Diagnosis, Evaluation, and Treatment of High Blood Pressure in Children and Adolescents. NIH Publication No. 05-5267. NHLBI; revised May 2005.

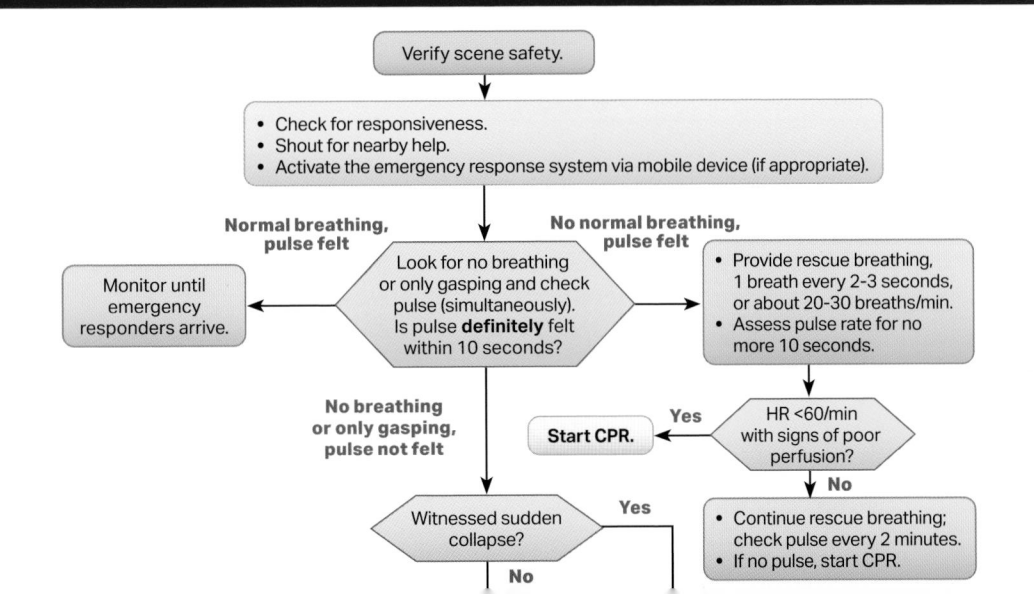

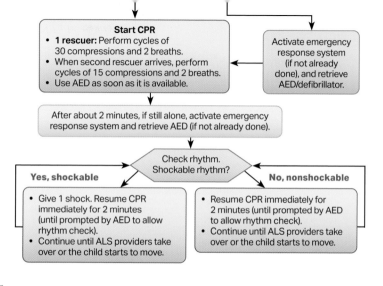

**Start CPR**
- **1 rescuer:** Perform cycles of 30 compressions and 2 breaths.
- When second rescuer arrives, perform cycles of 15 compressions and 2 breaths.
- Use AED as soon as it is available.

Activate emergency response system (if not already done), and retrieve AED/defibrillator.

After about 2 minutes, if still alone, activate emergency response system and retrieve AED (if not already done).

Check rhythm. Shockable rhythm?

**Yes, shockable**
- Give 1 shock. Resume CPR immediately for 2 minutes (until prompted by AED to allow rhythm check).
- Continue until ALS providers take over or the child starts to move.

**No, nonshockable**
- Resume CPR immediately for 2 minutes (until prompted by AED to allow rhythm check).
- Continue until ALS providers take over or the child starts to move.

Abbreviations: AED, automated external defibrillator; ALS, advanced life support; CPR, cardiopulmonary resuscitation; HR, heart rate.

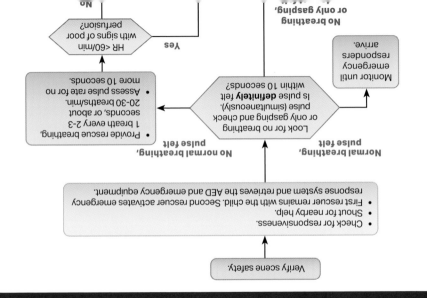

Verify scene safety.

- Check for responsiveness.
- Shout for nearby help.
- First rescuer remains with the child. Second rescuer activates emergency response system and retrieves the AED and emergency equipment.

Look for no breathing or only gasping and check pulse (simultaneously). Is pulse **definitely** felt within 10 seconds?

**Normal breathing, pulse felt**

Monitor until emergency responders arrive.

**No normal breathing, pulse felt**

- Provide rescue breathing, 1 breath every 2-3 seconds, or about 20-30 breaths/min.
- Assess pulse rate for no more 10 seconds.

HR <60/min with signs of poor perfusion?

No

Yes

**No breathing or only gasping**

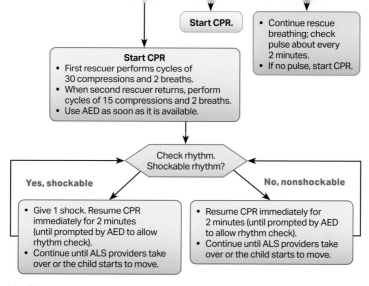

**Start CPR.**

- Continue rescue breathing; check pulse about every 2 minutes.
- If no pulse, start CPR.

**Start CPR**
- First rescuer performs cycles of 30 compressions and 2 breaths.
- When second rescuer returns, perform cycles of 15 compressions and 2 breaths.
- Use AED as soon as it is available.

Check rhythm.
Shockable rhythm?

**Yes, shockable**

**No, nonshockable**

- Give 1 shock. Resume CPR immediately for 2 minutes (until prompted by AED to allow rhythm check).
- Continue until ALS providers take over or the child starts to move.

- Resume CPR immediately for 2 minutes (until prompted by AED to allow rhythm check).
- Continue until ALS providers take over or the child starts to move.

Abbreviations: AED, automated external defibrillator; ALS, advanced life support; CPR, cardiopulmonary resuscitation; HR, heart rate.

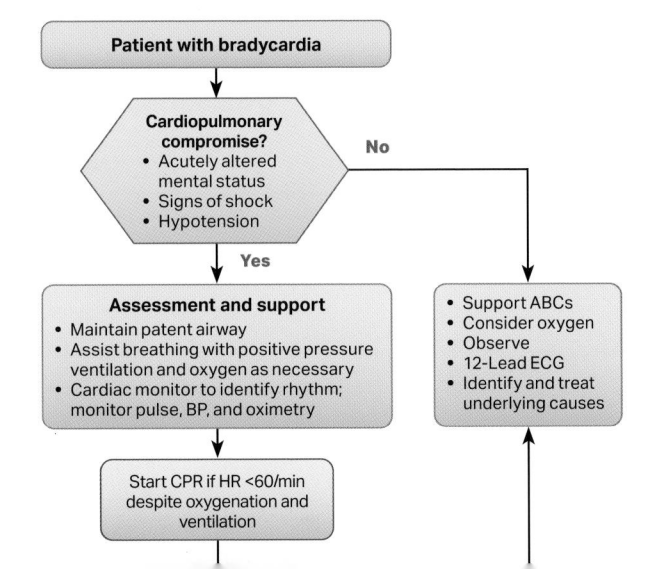

**Patient with bradycardia**

**Cardiopulmonary compromise?**
- Acutely altered mental status
- Signs of shock
- Hypotension

No

Yes

**Assessment and support**
- Maintain patent airway
- Assist breathing with positive pressure ventilation and oxygen as necessary
- Cardiac monitor to identify rhythm; monitor pulse, BP, and oximetry

- Support ABCs
- Consider oxygen
- Observe
- 12-Lead ECG
- Identify and treat underlying causes

Start CPR if HR <60/min despite oxygenation and ventilation

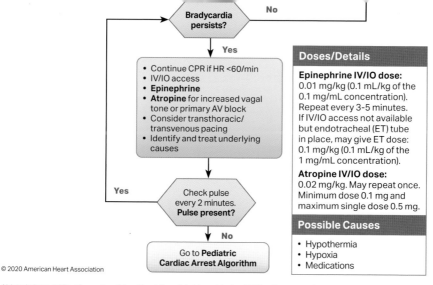

**Bradycardia persists?**

No

Yes

- Continue CPR if HR <60/min
- IV/IO access
- **Epinephrine**
- **Atropine** for increased vagal tone or primary AV block
- Consider transthoracic/transvenous pacing
- Identify and treat underlying causes

Yes

**Check pulse every 2 minutes. Pulse present?**

No

Go to **Pediatric Cardiac Arrest Algorithm**

### Doses/Details

**Epinephrine IV/IO dose:**
0.01 mg/kg (0.1 mL/kg of the 0.1 mg/mL concentration). Repeat every 3-5 minutes. If IV/IO access not available but endotracheal (ET) tube in place, may give ET dose: 0.1 mg/kg (0.1 mL/kg of the 1 mg/mL concentration).

**Atropine IV/IO dose:**
0.02 mg/kg. May repeat once. Minimum dose 0.1 mg and maximum single dose 0.5 mg.

### Possible Causes

- Hypothermia
- Hypoxia
- Medications

Abbreviations: ABCs, Airway-Breathing-Circulation; AV, atrioventricular; BP, blood pressure; CPR, cardiopulmonary resuscitation; ECG, electrocardiogram; ET, endotracheal; HR, heart rate; IO, intraosseous; IV, intravenous.

# Pediatric Cardiac Arrest Algorithm

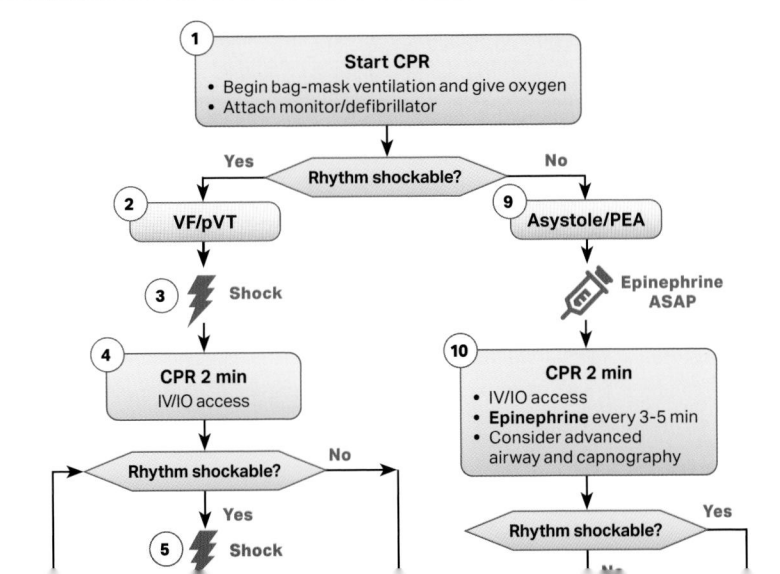

**1. Start CPR**
- Begin bag-mask ventilation and give oxygen
- Attach monitor/defibrillator

**Rhythm shockable?**

Yes → **2. VF/pVT**

No → **9. Asystole/PEA**

**3. Shock**

Epinephrine ASAP

**4. CPR 2 min**
IV/IO access

**10. CPR 2 min**
- IV/IO access
- **Epinephrine** every 3-5 min
- Consider advanced airway and capnography

**Rhythm shockable?**

No →

Yes → **5. Shock**

**Rhythm shockable?**

Yes →

No →

## CPR Quality

- Push hard (≥⅓ of anteroposterior diameter of chest) and fast (100-120/min) and allow complete chest recoil
- Minimize interruptions in compressions
- Change compressor every 2 minutes, or sooner if fatigued
- If no advanced airway, 15:2 compression-ventilation ratio
- If advanced airway, provide continuous compressions and give a breath every 2-3 seconds

## Shock Energy for Defibrillation

- First shock 2 J/kg
- Second shock 4 J/kg
- Subsequent shocks ≥4 J/kg, maximum 10 J/kg or adult dose

## Drug Therapy

- **Epinephrine IV/IO dose:**
  0.01 mg/kg (0.1 mL/kg of the 0.1 mg/mL concentration). Max dose 1 mg. Repeat every 3-5 minutes.
  If no IV/IO access, may give endotracheal dose: 0.1 mg/kg (0.1 mL/kg of the 1 mg/mL concentration)

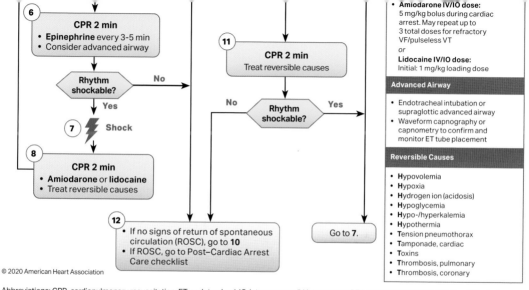

**6**

**CPR 2 min**
- **Epinephrine** every 3-5 min
- Consider advanced airway

**Rhythm shockable?** → No

↓ Yes

**7** ⚡ **Shock**

**8**

**CPR 2 min**
- **Amiodarone** or **lidocaine**
- Treat reversible causes

**11**

**CPR 2 min**
Treat reversible causes

No ← **Rhythm shockable?** → Yes

**12**
- If no signs of return of spontaneous circulation (ROSC), go to **10**
- If ROSC, go to Post–Cardiac Arrest Care checklist

Go to **7.**

- **Amiodarone IV/IO dose:**
5 mg/kg bolus during cardiac arrest. May repeat up to 3 total doses for refractory VF/pulseless VT

*or*

**Lidocaine IV/IO dose:**
Initial: 1 mg/kg loading dose

**Advanced Airway**

- Endotracheal intubation or supraglottic advanced airway
- Waveform capnography or capnometry to confirm and monitor ET tube placement

**Reversible Causes**

- **H**ypovolemia
- **H**ypoxia
- **H**ydrogen ion (acidosis)
- **H**ypoglycemia
- **H**ypo-/hyperkalemia
- **H**ypothermia
- **T**ension pneumothorax
- **T**amponade, cardiac
- **T**oxins
- **T**hrombosis, pulmonary
- **T**hrombosis, coronary

© 2020 American Heart Association

Abbreviations: CPR, cardiopulmonary resuscitation; ET, endotracheal; IO, intraosseous; IV, intravenous; PEA, pulseless electrical activity; pVT, pulseless ventricular tachycardia; ROSC, return of spontaneous circulation; VF, ventricular fibrillation.

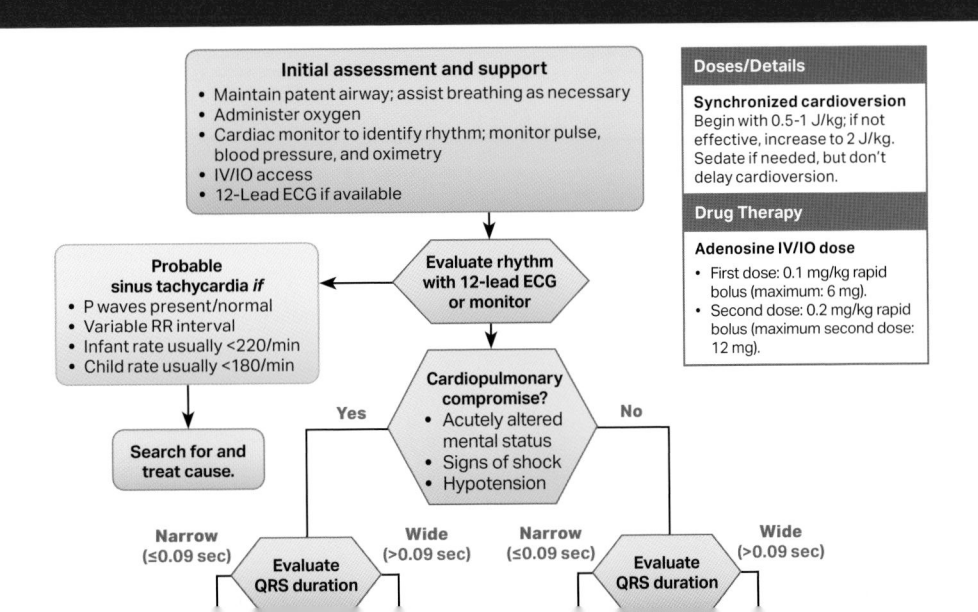

**Initial assessment and support**
- Maintain patent airway; assist breathing as necessary
- Administer oxygen
- Cardiac monitor to identify rhythm; monitor pulse, blood pressure, and oximetry
- IV/IO access
- 12-Lead ECG if available

**Doses/Details**

**Synchronized cardioversion**
Begin with 0.5-1 J/kg; if not effective, increase to 2 J/kg. Sedate if needed, but don't delay cardioversion.

**Drug Therapy**

**Adenosine IV/IO dose**
- First dose: 0.1 mg/kg rapid bolus (maximum: 6 mg).
- Second dose: 0.2 mg/kg rapid bolus (maximum second dose: 12 mg).

**Evaluate rhythm with 12-lead ECG or monitor**

**Probable sinus tachycardia if**
- P waves present/normal
- Variable RR interval
- Infant rate usually <220/min
- Child rate usually <180/min

**Search for and treat cause.**

**Cardiopulmonary compromise?**
- Acutely altered mental status
- Signs of shock
- Hypotension

Yes     No

**Narrow (≤0.09 sec)**    **Evaluate QRS duration**    **Wide (>0.09 sec)**    **Narrow (≤0.09 sec)**    **Evaluate QRS duration**    **Wide (>0.09 sec)**

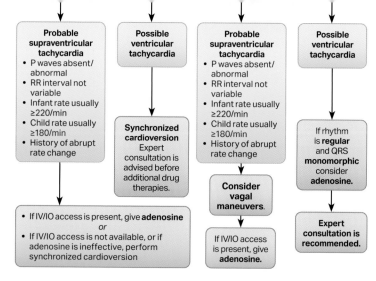

**Probable supraventricular tachycardia**
- P waves absent/abnormal
- RR interval not variable
- Infant rate usually ≥220/min
- Child rate usually ≥180/min
- History of abrupt rate change

**Possible ventricular tachycardia**

**Synchronized cardioversion**
Expert consultation is advised before additional drug therapies.

**Probable supraventricular tachycardia**
- P waves absent/abnormal
- RR interval not variable
- Infant rate usually ≥220/min
- Child rate usually ≥180/min
- History of abrupt rate change

**Consider vagal maneuvers**.

**Possible ventricular tachycardia**

If rhythm is **regular** and QRS **monomorphic** consider **adenosine**.

- If IV/IO access is present, give **adenosine**
  *or*
- If IV/IO access is not available, or if adenosine is ineffective, perform synchronized cardioversion

If IV/IO access is present, give **adenosine**.

**Expert consultation is recommended.**

Abbreviations: ECG, electrocardiogram; HR, heart rate; IO, intraosseous; IV, intravenous.

# Steps for Pediatric Defibrillation and Cardioversion

## Manual Defibrillation (for Ventricular Fibrillation or Pulseless Ventricular Tachycardia)

Continue CPR without interruptions during all steps until the defibrillator is fully charged. Minimize interval between the last compression and shock delivery (do not deliver breaths between the last compression and shock delivery).

1. Turn on defibrillator.
2. Set lead switch to paddles (or lead I, II, or III if monitor leads are used).
3. Select adhesive pads or paddles; use the largest pads or paddles that can fit on the patient's chest without touching each other.
4. If using paddles, apply conductive gel or paste. Be sure cables are attached to defibrillator.
5. Position the adhesive pads on the patient's chest: right anterior chest wall and left axillary positions. If using paddles, apply firm pressure. If patient has an implanted pacemaker, do not place the pads/ paddles directly over the device. Be sure that paddles are not placed on a nitroglycerin sheet.

## Cardioversion (for Unstable Supraventricular Tachycardia or Ventricular Tachycardia With a Pulse)

Consider expert consultation for suspected ventricular tachycardia (VT).

1. Turn on defibrillator.
2. Set lead switch to paddles (or lead I, II, or III if monitor leads are used).
3. Select adhesive pads to paddles. Use the largest pads or paddles that can fit on the patient's chest without touching each other.
4. If using paddles, apply conductive gel or paste. Be sure cables are attached to defibrillator.
5. Consider sedation.
6. Select *synchronized* mode.
7. Look for markers on R waves indicating that sync mode is operative. If necessary, adjust monitor gain until sync markers occur with each R wave.
8. Select energy dose:
   Initial dose: 0.5 to 1 J/kg
   Subsequent doses: 2 J/kg

**6.** Select energy dose:

**Initial dose:** 2 J/kg

**Subsequent doses:** 4 J/kg or higher (not to exceed 10 J/kg or standard adult dose)

**7.** Announce "Charging defibrillator," and press charge on defibrillator controls or apex paddle. Continue chest compressions during charging unless charging occurs immediately.

**8.** When defibrillator is fully charged, state a firm chant, such as "I am going to shock on three." Then count. This chant can be shortened to "Clear for shock." (Continue chest compressions until this announcement.)

**9.** After confirming all personnel are clear of the patient, press the Shock button on the defibrillator or press the 2 paddle *discharge* buttons simultaneously.

**10.** Immediately after shock delivery, resume CPR beginning with compressions for about 5 cycles (about 2 minutes), and then recheck rhythm. Minimize interruptions to compressions.

**9.** Announce "Charging defibrillator," and press Charge on the defibrillator controls or apex paddle.

**10.** When the defibrillator is fully charged, firmly state, "I am going to shock on 3." Then count and say, "All clear!"

**11.** After confirming all personnel are clear of the patient, press the Shock button on the defibrillator, or press both paddle discharge buttons simultaneously. Hold the paddles in place until a shock is delivered.

**12.** Check the monitor. If tachycardia persists, increase energy and prepare to attempt cardioversion again.

**13.** Reset the sync mode after each synchronized cardioversion because most defibrillators default to unsynchronized mode after synchronized shock delivery. This default allows an immediate defibrillation (nonsynchronized) shock if the cardioversion produces ventricular fibrillation.

*Note*: If ventricular fibrillation develops, immediately begin CPR, and prepare to deliver an unsynchronized shock as soon as possible (see Manual Defibrillation).

| Managing Respiratory Emergencies Flowchart | | |
|---|---|---|
| • Airway positioning<br>• Suction as needed | • Oxygen<br>• Pulse oximetry | • ECG monitor as indicated<br>• BLS as indicated |
| **Upper airway obstruction**<br>**Specific management for selected conditions** | | |
| **Croup** | **Anaphylaxis** | **Aspiration foreign body** |
| • Nebulized epinephrine<br>• Corticosteroids | • IM epinephrine (or autoinjector)<br>• Albuterol<br>• Antihistamines<br>• Corticosteroids | • Allow position of comfort<br>• Specialty consultation |
| **Lower airway obstruction**<br>**Specific management for selected conditions** | | |
| **Bronchiolitis** | **Asthma** | |
| • Nasal suctioning<br>• Consider bronchodilator trial | • Albuterol ± ipratropium<br>• Corticosteroids<br>• Magnesium sulfate | • IM epinephrine (if severe)<br>• Terbutaline |

*(continued)*

| Managing Respiratory Emergencies Flowchart | |
|---|---|
| **Lung tissue disease**<br>**Specific management for selected conditions** | |
| **Pneumonia/pneumonitis**<br>**Infectious, chemical, aspiration** | **Pulmonary edema**<br>**Cardiogenic or noncardiogenic (ARDS)** |
| • Albuterol<br>• Antibiotics (as indicated)<br>• Consider noninvasive or invasive ventilatory support with PEEP | • Consider noninvasive or invasive ventilatory support with PEEP<br>• Consider vasoactive support<br>• Consider diuretic |

| Disordered control of breathing<br>Specific management for selected conditions | | |
|---|---|---|
| **Increased ICP** | **Poisoning/overdose** | **Neuromuscular disease** |
| • Avoid hypoxemia<br>• Avoid hypercarbia<br>• Avoid hyperthermia<br>• Avoid hypotension | • Antidote (if available)<br>• Contact poison control | • Consider noninvasive or invasive ventilatory support |

Abbreviations: ARDS, acute respiratory distress syndrome; CPAP, continuous positive airway pressure; ECG, electrocardiographic; ICP, intracranial pressure; IM, intramuscular; PEEP, positive end-expiratory pressure.

## Pre-event Equipment Checklist for Endotracheal Intubation

- ☐ Universal precautions (gloves, mask, eye protection)
- ☐ Cardiac monitor, pulse oximeter, and blood pressure monitoring device
- ☐ End-tidal $CO_2$ detector or exhaled $CO_2$ capnography (or esophageal detector device, if appropriate)
- ☐ Intravenous and intraosseous infusion equipment
- ☐ Oxygen supply, bag-mask (appropriate size)
- ☐ Oral/tracheal suction equipment (appropriate size); confirm that it is working
- ☐ Oral and nasopharyngeal airways (appropriate size)
- ☐ Endotracheal tubes with stylets (all sizes) and sizes 0.5 mm (internal diameter) above and below anticipated size for patient; it is reasonable to choose cuffed over uncuffed ETTs.
- ☐ Laryngoscope (curved and straight blades) and/or video laryngoscope; backup laryngoscope available
- ☐ 3-, 5-, and 10-mL syringes to test inflate endotracheal tube balloon
- ☐ Adhesive/cloth tape or commercial endotracheal tube holder to secure tube
- ☐ Towel or pad to align airway by placing under head or torso
- ☐ Specialty equipment as needed for difficult airway management or anticipated complications (supraglottic, transtracheal, and/or cricothyrotomy)

## RSI Protocol for PALS

| Pre-event preparation | 1. Obtain brief medical history and perform focused physical examination.<br>2. Prepare equipment, monitors, personnel, medications.<br>3. If neck injury not suspected: place in sniffing position. If neck injury suspected: stabilize cervical spine. |
|---|---|
| Preoxygenate | 4. Preoxygenate with $FiO_2$ of 100% by mask (nonrebreather preferred). If ventilatory assistance is necessary, ventilate gently. |
| Premedicate/sedate | 5. Although no longer recommended routinely, consideration of atropine (for excessive secretions and/or high vagal tone) or glycopyrrolate (for excessive secretions) may be considered. |
| Pharmacologic sedation/anesthesia/ neuromuscular blockade and protection/positioning | 6. Administer sedation/anesthesia by IV push.<br>7. Give neuromuscular blocking agent by IV push.<br>8. Assess for apnea, jaw relaxation, and absence of movement (patient sufficiently relaxed to proceed with intubation). |
| Placement of endotracheal tube | 9. Perform endotracheal intubation. If during intubation oxygen saturation is inadequate, stop laryngoscopy and start ventilation with bag-mask. Monitor pulse oximetry and ensure adequate oxygen saturation. Reattempt intubation. Once intubated, inflate cuff (if cuffed tracheal tube is used) to minimal occlusive volume. Be prepared to place rescue airway (eg, supraglottic airway) if intubation attempts are unsuccessful. |
| Placement confirmation | 10. Confirm placement of endotracheal tube by<br> • Monitoring $O_2$ saturation and exhaled $CO_2$ levels (capnometry or waveform capnography)<br> • Direct visualization of ETT passing through vocal cords<br> • Chest rise/fall with each ventilation (bilateral)<br> • 5-point auscultation: anterior chest L and R, midaxillary line L and R, and over the epigastrium (no breath sounds over epigastrium); look for tube condensation<br> • Using end-tidal $CO_2$ detector (or esophageal detector device, if appropriate) |
| Postintubation management | 11. Prevent dislodgement:<br> • Secure ETT with adhesive/cloth tape or commercial ETT holder<br> • Continue cervical spine immobilization (if needed)<br> • Continue sedation; add paralytics if necessary |

Abbreviations: ETT, endotracheal tube; IV, intravenous; IO, intraosseous.

## Pharmacologic Agents Used for Rapid Sequence Intubation in Children

| Drug | IV/IO Dose* | Onset | Duration | Side Effects | Comments |
|------|-------------|-------|----------|--------------|----------|
| **Premedication Agents** | | | | | |
| **Atropine** | 0.01-0.02 mg/ kg (maximum: 0.5 mg) | 1-2 min | 2-4 hours | Tachycardia, agitation | Antisialagogue Inhibits bradycardic response to hypoxemia laryngoscopy, and succinylcholine May cause pupil dilation |
| **Glycopyrrolate** | 0.005-0.01 mg/ kg (maximum: 0.2 mg) | 1-2 min | 4-6 hours | Tachycardia | Antisialagogue Inhibits bradycardic response to hypoxemia |
| **Lidocaine** | 1-2 mg/kg | 1-2 min | 10-20 min | Myocardial and CNS depression with high doses Seizures | May decrease ICP during RSI May decrease pain on propofol injection |

*(continued)*

| Drug | IV/IO Dose* | Onset | Duration | Side Effects | Comments |
|---|---|---|---|---|---|
| **Sedative Agents** | | | | | |
| **Etomidate** | 0.2-0.4 mg/kg | <1 min | 5-10 min | Myoclonic activity Cortisol suppression | Ultrashort acting No analgesic properties Decreases cerebral metabolic rate and ICP Generally maintains hemodynamic stability Avoid routine use in patients with suspected septic shock (inhibits cortisol synthesis) |
| **Fentanyl citrate** | 2-5 mcg/kg | 1-3 min | 30-60 min | Chest wall rigidity possible with high-dose rapid infusions | Minimum histamine release May lower blood pressure (especially with higher doses or in conjunction with midazolam) |
| **Ketamine** | 1-2 mg/kg | 30-60 sec | 10-20 min | Hypertension, tachycardia Increased secretions and laryngospasm Emergence reactions/ hallucinations | Dissociative anesthetic agent Limited respiratory depression Bronchodilator May cause myocardial depression in catecholamine-depleted patients |

*(continued)*

| Drug | IV/IO Dose* | Onset | Duration | Side Effects | Comments |
|---|---|---|---|---|---|
| **Sedative Agents** | | | | | |
| **Midazolam** | 0.1-0.3 mg/kg (maximum single dose: 10 mg) | 2-5 min | 15-30 min | Hypotension | Hypotension exacerbated in combination with narcotics and barbiturates No analgesic properties Excellent amnestic |
| **Diazepam** | 0.2-0.3 mg/kg (maximum single dose: 10 mg) | 1-3 min | 20-40 min | | |
| **Propofol** | 1-2 mg/kg (up to 3 mg/kg in children 6 months to 5 years of age) | <1 min | 5-10 min | Hypotension, especially in patients with inadequate intravascular volume Pain on infusion | No analgesic properties Very short duration of action Less airway reactivity than barbiturates Decreases cerebral metabolic rate and ICP Lidocaine may decrease infusion pain Not recommended in patients with egg/soy allergy |

(continued)

| Drug | IV/IO Dose* | Onset | Duration | Side Effects | Comments |
|---|---|---|---|---|---|
| **Neuromuscular Blocking Agents** | | | | | |
| **Succinylcholine** | 1-1.5 mg/kg for children; 2 mg/kg for infants | 45-60 sec | 4-6 min | May cause rhabdomyolysis; rise in intracranial, intraocular, intragastric pressure; life-threatening hyperkalemia | Depolarizing muscle relaxant Rapid onset, short duration of action Avoid in renal failure, burns, crush injuries after 48 hours, muscular dystrophy and other neuromuscular diseases, hyperkalemia, or family history of malignant hyperthermia Do *not* use to maintain paralysis |
| **Vecuronium** | 0.1-0.3 mg/kg | 3-5 min | 30-60 min | Minimal cardiovascular side effects | Nondepolarizing agent The higher the dose, the quicker the onset of action and the longer the duration |
| **Rocuronium** | 0.6-1.2 mg/kg | 30-60 sec | Infant 3-12 months: 40 min Children 1-12 years: 26-30 min | Minimal cardiovascular side effects | Nondepolarizing agent Rapid onset of action |

Abbreviations: ICP, intracranial pressure; IO, intraosseous; IV, intravenous; RSI, rapid sequence intubation.

*Doses provided are guidelines only. Actual dosing may vary depending on patient's clinical status.

**1**

## Identify signs of septic shock

- Altered **mental status** (irritability or decreased level of consciousness)
- Altered **heart rate** (tachycardia or, less commonly, bradycardia)
- Altered **temperature** (fever or hypothermia)
- Altered **perfusion** (prolonged or "flash" capillary refill; cool or very warm extremities; plethoric appearance, mottled color or pallor; possible ecchymosis or purpura; decreased urine output)
- **Hypotension:** May or may not be present

*Immediate (10-15 min)*

**2**

## Initial stabilization

- Support A-B-Cs.
- Monitor heart rate, blood pressure, and pulse oximetry.
- Establish IV/IO access.
- Fluid boluses: Give 10-20 mL/kg isotonic crystalloid boluses (10 mL/kg for neonates and those with pre-existing cardiovascular compromise). Assess carefully after each bolus.

**3**

## Within first hour

- Draw blood for culture and additional laboratory studies, including glucose and calcium and do not delay antibiotic or fluid therapy.
- Antibiotics: Give broad spectrum antibiotics.
- Assess carefully after each fluid bolus. Repeat fluid boluses as needed to treat shock. Stop if rales, respiratory distress, or hepatomegaly develops.
- Give antipyretics if needed

**Goals of therapy:** Improved mental status, normalization of heart rate and temperature, adequate systolic and diastolic blood pressure, improved perfusion (see 1)

*First hour*

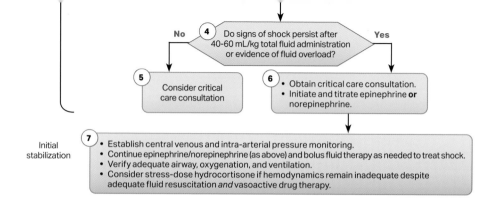

**No** ④ Do signs of shock persist after 40-60 mL/kg total fluid administration or evidence of fluid overload? **Yes**

⑤ Consider critical care consultation

⑥ • Obtain critical care consultation.
• Initiate and titrate epinephrine **or** norepinephrine.

**Initial stabilization**

⑦ • Establish central venous and intra-arterial pressure monitoring.
• Continue epinephrine/norepinephrine (as above) and bolus fluid therapy as needed to treat shock.
• Verify adequate airway, oxygenation, and ventilation.
• Consider stress-dose hydrocortisone if hemodynamics remain inadequate despite adequate fluid resuscitation *and* vasoactive drug therapy.

Brierley J, Carcillo JA, Choong K, et al. Clinical practice parameters for hemodynamic support of pediatric and neonatal septic shock: 2007 update from the American College of Critical Care Medicine. *Crit Care Med.* 2009;37(2):666-688. Kissoon N, Orr RA, Carcillo JA. Updated American College of Critical Care Medicine—pediatric advanced life support guidelines for management of pediatric and neonatal septic shock: relevance to the emergency care clinician. *Pediatr Emerg Care.* 2010;26(11):867-869.

Abbreviations: IO, intraosseous; IV, intravenous.

## Glasgow Coma Scale*

| Score | Child | Infant |
|:---:|---|---|
| **Eye opening** | | |
| 4 | Spontaneously | Spontaneously |
| 3 | To verbal command | To shout, speech |
| 2 | To pain | To pain |
| 1 | No response | No response |
| **Best motor response** | | |
| 6 | Obeys commands | Spontaneous movements |
| 5 | Localizes pain | Withdraws to touch |
| 4 | Flexion-appropriate withdraw | Flexion-appropriate withdraw |
| 3 | Flexion-abnormal (decorticate rigidity) | Flexion-abnormal (decorticate rigidity) |
| 2 | Extension (decerebrate rigidity) | Extension (decerebrate rigidity) |
| 1 | No response | No response |

(continued)

| Score | Child | Infant |
|:---:|---|---|
| **Best verbal response** | | |
| 5 | Oriented and converses | Smiles, coos, and babbles |
| 4 | Disoriented, confused | Cries but is consolable |
| 3 | Inappropriate words | Persistent, inappropriate crying and/or screaming |
| 2 | Incomprehensible sounds | Moans, grunts to pain |
| 1 | No response | No response |
| **Total = 3 to 15** | | |

*Score is the sum of the individual scores from eye opening, best motor response, and best verbal response, using age-specific criteria. GCS score of 13 to 15 indicates mild head injury; GCS score of 9 to 12 indicates moderate head injury; and GCS score of ≤8 indicates severe head injury.

Modified from James HE, Trauner DA. The Glasgow Coma Score and Modified Coma Score for Infants. In: James HE, Anas NG, Perkin RM, eds. Brain Insults in Infants and Children: Pathophysiology and Management. Orlando, FL: Grune & Stratton Inc; 1985:179-182, copyright Elsevier.

# Systemic Responses to Blood Loss in Pediatric Patients

| System | Mild Blood Volume Loss (<30%) | Moderate Blood Volume Loss (30%-45%) | Severe Blood Volume Loss (>45%) |
|---|---|---|---|
| Cardiovascular | Increased heart rate; weak, thready peripheral pulses; normal systolic blood pressure (80-90 + 2 × age in years); normal pulse pressure | Markedly increased heart rate; weak, thready central pulses; absent peripheral pulses; low normal systolic blood pressure (70-80 + 2 × age in years); narrowed pulse pressure | Tachycardia followed by bradycardia; very weak or absent central pulses; absent peripheral pulses; hypotension (<70 + 2 × age in years); narrowed pulse pressure (or undetectable diastolic blood pressure) |
| Central nervous system | Anxious; irritable; confused | Lethargic; dulled response to pain* | Comatose |
| Skin | Cool, mottled; prolonged capillary refill | Cyanotic; markedly prolonged capillary refill | Pale and cold |
| Urine output† | Low to very low | Minimal | None |

*A child's dulled response to pain with moderate blood loss may indicate a decreased response to IV catheter insertion.

†Monitor urine output after initial decompression by urinary catheter. Low normal is 2 mL/kg per hour (infant), 1.5 mL/kg per hour (younger child), 1 mL/kg per hour (older child), and 0.5 mL/kg per hour (adolescent). Intravenous contrast can falsely elevate urinary output.

Adaptation of the original table from American College of Surgeons. *Advanced Trauma Life Support® Student Course Manual*. 10th ed. American College

# Post–Cardiac Arrest Care Checklist

(continued)

| Components of Post–Cardiac Arrest Care | Check |
|---|:---:|
| **Oxygenation and ventilation** | |
| Measure oxygenation and target normoxemia 94%-99% (or child's normal/appropriate oxygen saturation). | ☐ |
| Measure and target PaCO$_2$ appropriate to the patient's underlying condition and limit exposure to severe hypercapnia or hypocapnia. | ☐ |
| **Hemodynamic monitoring** | |
| Set specific hemodynamic goals during post–cardiac arrest care and review daily. | ☐ |
| Monitor with cardiac telemetry. | ☐ |
| Monitor arterial blood pressure. | ☐ |
| Monitor serum lactate, urine output, and central venous oxygen saturation to help guide therapies. | ☐ |
| Use parenteral fluid bolus with or without inotropes or vasopressors to maintain a systolic blood pressure greater than the fifth percentile for age and sex. | ☐ |
| **Targeted temperature management (TTM)** | |
| Measure and continuously monitor core temperature. | ☐ |
| Prevent and treat fever immediately after arrest and during rewarming. | ☐ |
| If patient is comatose, apply TTM (32°C-34°C) followed by TTM (36°C-37.5°C) or only TTM (36°C-37.5°C). | ☐ |
| Prevent shivering. | ☐ |
| Monitor blood pressure and treat hypotension during rewarming. | ☐ |

| Components of Post–Cardiac Arrest Care | Check |
|---|---|
| **Neuromonitoring** | |
| If patient has encephalopathy and resources are available, monitor with continuous electroencephalogram. | ☐ |
| Treat seizures. | ☐ |
| Consider early brain imaging to diagnose treatable causes of cardiac arrest. | ☐ |
| **Electrolytes and glucose** | |
| Measure blood glucose and avoid hypoglycemia. | ☐ |
| Maintain electrolytes within normal ranges to avoid possible life-threatening arrhythmias. | ☐ |
| **Sedation** | |
| Treat with sedatives and anxiolytics. | ☐ |
| **Prognosis** | |
| Always consider multiple modalities (clinical and other) over any single predictive factor. | ☐ |
| Remember that assessments may be modified by TTM or induced hypothermia. | ☐ |
| Consider electroencephalogram in conjunction with other factors within the first 7 days after cardiac arrest. | ☐ |
| Consider neuroimaging such as magnetic resonance imaging during the first 7 days. | ☐ |

### Optimize Ventilation and Oxygenation

- Titrate $FiO_2$ to maintain oxyhemoglobin saturation 94%-99% (or as appropriate to the patient's condition); if possible, wean $FiO_2$ if saturation is 100%.
- Consider advanced airway placement and waveform capnography.
- If possible, target a $PCO_2$ that is appropriate for the patient's condition and limit exposure to severe hypercapnia or hypocapnia.

### Assess for and Treat Persistent Shock

- Identify and treat contributing factors.
- Consider 20 mL/kg IV/IO boluses of isotonic crystalloid. Consider smaller boluses (eg, 10 mL/kg) if poor cardiac function suspected.
- Consider the need for inotropic and/or vasopressor support for fluid-refractory shock.

$\longleftrightarrow$

### Possible Contributing Factors

**H**ypovolemia
**H**ypoxia
**H**ydrogen ion (acidosis)
**H**ypoglycemia
**H**ypo-/hyperkalemia
**H**ypothermia

**T**ension pneumothorax
**T**amponade, cardiac
**T**oxins
**T**hrombosis, pulmonary
**T**hrombosis, coronary
**T**rauma

### Estimation of Maintenance Fluid Requirements

- **Infants <10 kg:** 4 mL/kg per hour

  *Example:* For an 8-kg infant, estimated maintenance fluid rate
  = 4 mL/kg per hour × 8 kg
  = 32 mL per hour

- **Children 10-20 kg:** 4 mL/kg per hour for the first 10 kg + 2 mL/kg per hour for each kg above 10 kg

  *Example:* For a 15-kg child, estimated maintenance fluid rate
  = (4 mL/kg per hour × 10 kg)
  + (2 mL/kg per hour × 5 kg)
  = 40 mL/hour + 10 mL/hour
  = 50 mL/hour

- **Children >20 kg:** 4 mL/kg per hour for the first 10 kg + 2 mL/kg per hour for 11-20 kg + 1 mL/kg per hour for each kg above 20 kg

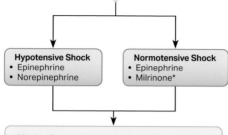

**Hypotensive Shock**
- Epinephrine
- Norepinephrine

**Normotensive Shock**
- Epinephrine
- Milrinone*

- Monitor for and treat agitation and seizures.
- Monitor for and treat hypoglycemia.
- Assess blood gas, serum electrolytes, and calcium.
- If patient remains comatose after resuscitation from cardiac arrest, maintain targeted temperature management, including aggressive treatment of fever.
- Consider consultation and patient transport to tertiary care center.

*Example.* For a 28-kg child, estimated maintenance fluid rate
= (4 mL/kg per hour × 10 kg)
  + (2 mL/kg per hour × 10 kg)
  + (1 mL/kg per hour × 8 kg)
= 40 mL per hour + 20 mL per hour
  + 8 mL per hour
= 68 mL per hour

After initial stabilization, adjust the rate and composition of intravenous fluids based on the patient's clinical condition and state of hydration. In general, provide a continuous infusion of a dextrose-containing solution for infants. Avoid hypotonic solutions in critically ill children; for most patients, use isotonic fluid such as normal saline (0.9% NaCl) or lactated Ringer's solution with or without dextrose, based on the child's clinical status.

*Milrinone can cause hypotension, so use and initiation of it should generally be reserved for those experienced with its use, initiation, and side effects (eg, ICU personnel).

Abbreviations: IO, intraosseous; IV, intravenous; ROSC, return of spontaneous circulation.

# Pediatric Resuscitation Supplies Based on Color-Coded Length-Based Resuscitation Tape

| Zone | 3 kg <3 mos | 4 kg <3 mos | 5 kg <3 mos | Pink 6–7 kg 3–5 mos | Red 8–9 kg 6–9 mos | Purple 10–11 kg 12–24 mos | Yellow 12–14 kg 2 years | White 15–18 kg 3–4 yrs | Blue 19–23 kg 5–6 yrs | Orange 24–29 kg 7–9 yrs | Green 30–36 kg 10–11 yrs |
|---|---|---|---|---|---|---|---|---|---|---|---|
| ETT uncuffed (mm) | 3.5 | 3.5 | 3.5 | 3.5 | 3.5 | 4.0 | 4.5 | 5.0 | 5.5 | N/A | N/A |
| ETT cuffed (mm) | 3.0 | 3.0 | 3.0 | 3.0 | 3.0 | 3.5 | 4.0 | 4.5 | 5.0 | 5.5 | 6.0 |
| Lip-tip (cm) | 9–9.5 | 9.5–10 | 9.5–10 | 10–10.5 | 10–10.5 | 11–12 | 12.5–13.5 | 14–15 | 15.5–16.5 | 17–18 | 18.5–19.5 |
| Suction (F) | 8 | 8 | 8 | 8 | 8 | 8 | 10 | 10 | 10 | 10 | 12 |
| L-scope blade | 1 straight | 1 straight | 1 straight | 1 straight | 1 straight | 1–1.5 straight | 2 straight/ curved | 2 straight/ curved | 2 straight/ curved | 2–3 straight/ curved | 2–3 straight/ curved |
| Stylet | 6F | 6F | 6F | 6F | 6F | 6F | 6F | 10F | 10F | 14F | 14F |
| OPA (mm) | 50 | 50 | 50 | 50 | 50 | 50 | 60 | 60 | 70 | 80 | 80 |
| NPA (F) | 14 | 14 | 14 | 14 | 14 | 18 | 20 | 22 | 24 | 26 | 26 |
| Bag-mask device (minimum mL) | 450 | 450 | 450 | 450 | 450 | 450 | 450 | 450–750 | 750–1000 | 750–1000 | 1000 |
| ETCO₂ detector | Ped | Ped | Ped | Ped | Ped | Ped | Ped | Adult | Adult | Adult | Adult |
| LMA | 1 | 1 | 1 | 1.5 | 1.5 | 2 | 2 | 2 | 2.5 | 2.5 | 3 |
| Tidal volume (mL) | 20–30 | 24–40 | 30–50 | 40–65 | 50–85 | 65–105 | 80–130 | 100–165 | 125–210 | 160–265 | 200–330 |
| Frequency | 20–25/min | 20–25/min | 20–25/min | 20–25/min | 20–25/min | 15–25/min | 15–25/min | 15–25/min | 12–20/min | 12–20/min | 12–20/min |

Abbreviations: ETCO₂, end-tidal carbon dioxide; ETT, endotracheal tube; F, French; LMA, laryngeal mask airway; NPA, nasopharyngeal airway; OPA, oropharyngeal airway; Ped, pediatric.

## Estimating Endotracheal Tube Size and Depth of Insertion

### Tube Size

Several formulas, such as the ones below, allow estimation of proper ETT size (internal diameter [i.d.]) for children 2 to 10 years of age, based on the child's age:

**Uncuffed endotracheal tube size** (mm i.d.) = (age in years/4)+4

During preparation for intubation, providers also should have ready at the bedside uncuffed endotracheal tubes 0.5 mm smaller and larger than that estimated from the above formula.

The formula for estimation of a cuffed endotracheal tube size is as follows:

**Cuffed endotracheal tube size** (mm i.d.) = (age in years/4)+3.5

Typical cuffed inflation pressure should be less than 20 to 25 cm $H_2O$.

---

### Depth of Insertion

The formula for estimation of depth of insertion (measured at the lip) can be estimated from the child's age or the tube size.

**Depth of insertion** (cm) for children older than 2 years of age = (age in years/2)+12

or

**Depth of insertion** = tube i.d. (mm)×3

**Confirm placement with both device (eg, exhaled $CO_2$ detector) and clinical assessment (eg, breath sounds, chest expansion). Watch for marker on endotracheal tube at vocal cords.**

## Administration Notes

**Peripheral intravenous (IV):** Resuscitation drugs administered via peripheral IV catheter should be followed by a bolus of at least 5 mL NS to move drug into central circulation.

**Intraosseous (IO):** All drugs or all medications that can be administered by IV route can be administered by IO route. They should be followed by a bolus of at least 5 mL NS to move drug into central circulation.

**Endotracheal:** Although some drugs can be administered endotracheally, IV/IO administration is preferred because it provides more reliable drug delivery and pharmacologic effect. Drugs that can be administered by endotracheal route are noted in the table below. Optimal endotracheal doses have not yet been established. Doses given by endotracheal route should generally be higher than standard IV doses. For infants and children, dilute the medication with NS to a volume of 3-5 mL, instill in the endotracheal tube, and follow with flush of 3-5 mL. Provide 5 positive-pressure breaths after medication is instilled.

| Drug/Therapy | Indications/Precautions | Pediatric Dosage |
|---|---|---|
| **Adenosine** | **Indications**<br>Drug of choice for treatment of symptomatic SVT<br><br>**Precautions**<br>• Very short half-life<br>• Limited adult data suggest need to reduce dose in patients taking carbamazepine and dipyridamole<br>• Less effective (larger doses may be required) in patients taking theophylline or caffeine | **IV/IO Administration**<br>• First dose<br>  – 0.1 mg/kg IV/IO rapid push<br>  – Maximum dose: 6 mg<br>• Second dose<br>  – 0.2 mg/kg IV/IO rapid push<br>  – Maximum dose: 12 mg<br>• Follow immediately with 5-10 mL NS flush<br>• Continuous ECG monitoring<br><br>**Injection Technique**<br>• Record rhythm strip during administration<br>• Draw up adenosine dose in one syringe and flush in another. Attach both syringes to the same or immediately adjacent IV injection ports nearest patient, with adenosine closest to patient<br>• Clamp IV tubing above injection port<br>• Push IV adenosine as quickly as possible (1-3 seconds)<br>• While maintaining pressure on adenosine plunger, push NS flush as rapidly as possible after adenosine<br>• Unclamp IV tubing |

| Drug/Therapy | Indications/Precautions | Pediatric Dosage |
|---|---|---|
| **Albuterol**<br><br>Nebulized solution:<br>0.5% (5 mg/mL)<br><br>Prediluted nebulized solution:<br>0.63 mg/3 mL NS,<br>1.25 mg/3 mL NS,<br>2.5 mg/3 mL NS<br>(0.083%)<br><br>MDI: 90 mcg/puff | **Indications**<br>Bronchodilator, β$_2$-adrenergic agent<br><br>• Asthma<br>• Anaphylaxis (bronchospasm)<br>• Hyperkalemia | **For Asthma, Anaphylaxis (Mild to Moderate), Hyperkalemia**<br>• **MDI (every 20 minutes)**<br>  – 4-8 puffs (inhalation) PRN with spacer<br>• **Nebulizer (every 20 minutes)**<br>  – Weight <20 kg: 2.5 mg/dose (inhalation)<br>  – Weight >20 kg: 5 mg/dose (inhalation)<br><br>**For Asthma, Anaphylaxis (Severe)**<br>• **Continuous nebulizer**<br>  – 0.5 mg/kg per hour continuous inhalation (maximum dose 20 mg/h)<br>• **MDI (recommended if intubated)**<br>  – 4-8 puffs (inhalation) via endotracheal tube every 20 minutes PRN or with spacer if not intubated |
| **Alprostadil (PGE₁)**<br>(see *Prostaglandin E₁*) | | |

## Amiodarone

### Indications

Can be used for treatment of atrial and ventricular arrhythmias in children, particularly ectopic atrial tachycardia, junctional ectopic tachycardia, and ventricular tachycardia/ventricular fibrillation

### Precautions

- May produce hypotension; may prolong QT interval and increase propensity for polymorphic ventricular arrhythmias. Therefore, routine administration in combination with procainamide is not recommended without expert consultation
- Use with caution if hepatic failure is present
- Terminal elimination is extremely long (elimination half-life with long-term oral dosing is up to 40 days)

### For Refractory VF, Pulseless VT

- 5 mg/kg IV/IO bolus; can repeat the 5 mg/kg IV/IO bolus up to total dose of 15 mg/kg (2.2 g in adolescents) IV per 24 hours
- Maximum single dose: 300 mg

### For Poor Perfusing Supraventricular and Ventricular Arrhythmias

Loading dose: 5 mg/kg IV/IO over 20-60 minutes (maximum single dose: 300 mg); can repeat to maximum of 15 mg/kg (2.2 g in adolescents) per day IV

| Drug/Therapy | Indications/Precautions | Pediatric Dosage |
|---|---|---|
| **Atropine Sulfate**<br>Can be given by endotracheal tube | **Indications**<br>• Symptomatic bradycardia (usually secondary to vagal stimulation)<br>• Toxins/overdose (organophosphate and carbamate poisoning)<br>• Rapid sequence intubation (RSI): ie, age < 1 year, age 1–5 years receiving succinylcholine, age > 5 years receiving second dose of succinylcholine<br><br>**Precautions**<br>• Contraindicated in angle-closure glaucoma, tachyarrhythmias, and thyrotoxicosis<br>• Drug blocks bradycardic response to hypoxia. Monitor with pulse oximetry. | **Symptomatic Bradycardia**<br>• **IV/IO:** 0.02 mg/kg<br>  – Maximum single dose: 0.5 mg<br>  – May repeat dose once in 3–5 minutes<br>  – Maximum total dose for child: 1 mg; for adolescent: 3 mg<br>  – Larger doses may be needed for organophosphate poisoning<br>• **Endotracheal:** 0.04–0.06 mg/kg<br><br>**Toxins/Overdose (Organophosphate and Carbamate Poisoning)**<br>• < 12 years: 0.05 mg/kg IV/IO initially; then repeated and doubling the dose every 5 minutes until muscarinic symptoms reverse<br>• ≥ 12 years: 1 mg IV/IO initially; then repeated and doubling the dose every 5 minutes until muscarinic symptoms reverse<br><br>**RSI**<br>• **IV/IO:** 0.01–0.02 mg/kg (maximum dose: 0.5 mg)<br>• **IM:** 0.02 mg/kg |

## Calcium Chloride

10% = 100 mg/mL = 27.2 mg/mL elemental calcium

### Indications

- Treatment of documented or suspected conditions
  - Hypocalcemia
  - Hyperkalemia
- Consider for treatment of
  - Hypermagnesemia
  - Calcium channel blocker overdose

### Precautions

- Routine calcium administration is not recommended in pediatric cardiac arrest and may cause overall harm to the patient (and may contribute to cellular injury)
- Not recommended for routine treatment of asystole or PEA
- Rapid IV administration may cause hypotension, bradycardia, or asystole (particularly if patient is receiving digoxin)
- Precipitation risk: Do not mix with or infuse immediately before or after sodium bicarbonate without intervening flush

### IV/IO Administration

- 20 mg/kg slow IV/IO push
- May repeat if documented or suspected clinical indication persists (eg, toxicologic problem)
- Central venous administration preferred if available

# Pediatric Advanced Life Support Drugs

| Drug/Therapy | Indications/Precautions | Pediatric Dosage |
|---|---|---|
| **Calcium Gluconate**<br>10% = 100 mg/mL =<br>9 mg/mL elemental<br>calcium | **Indications**<br>• Treatment of documented or suspected conditions<br>  – Hypocalcemia<br>  – Hyperkalemia<br>• Consider for treatment of<br>  – Hypermagnesemia<br>  – Calcium channel blocker overdose<br><br>**Precautions**<br>• Routine calcium administration is not recommended for pediatric cardiac arrest and may cause overall harm to the patient (may contribute to cellular injury)<br>• Not recommended for routine treatment of asystole or PEA<br>• Rapid IV administration may cause hypotension, bradycardia, or asystole (particularly if patient is receiving digoxin)<br>• Do not mix with or infuse immediately before or after sodium bicarbonate without intervening flush | **IV/IO Administration**<br>• 60 mg/kg (0.6 mL/kg) slow IV/IO push<br>• May repeat if documented or suspected clinical indication persists (eg, toxicologic problem)<br>• Central venous administration preferred if available |

| *Corticosteroids* | **Precautions**<br>May cause hypertension, hyperglycemia, and increased risk of gastric bleeding | |
| --- | --- | --- |
| **Dexamethasone** | **Indications**<br>• Croup<br>• Asthma | *Dexamethasone*<br>**For Croup**<br>0.6 mg/kg PO/IM/IV×1 dose<br>(maximum dose: 16 mg)<br><br>**For Asthma**<br>0.6 mg/kg PO/IM/IV every 24 hours<br>(maximum dose: 16 mg) |
| **Hydrocortisone** | **Indications**<br>Treatment of adrenal insufficiency (may be associated with septic shock) | *Hydrocortisone*<br>**Adrenal Insufficiency**<br>2 mg/kg IV/IO bolus<br>(maximum dose: 100 mg) |
| **Methylprednisolone** | **Indications**<br>• Asthma (status asthmaticus)<br>• Anaphylactic shock | *Methylprednisolone*<br>Use sodium succinate salt.<br>**Status Asthmaticus, Anaphylactic Shock**<br>• Load: 2 mg/kg IV/IO/IM (maximum: 60 mg)<br>• Maintenance: 0.5 mg/kg IV every 6 hours or 1 mg/kg every 12 hours up to 120 mg/day |

# Pediatric Advanced Life Support Drugs

| Drug/Therapy | Indications/Precautions | Pediatric Dosage |
|---|---|---|
| **Epinephrine**<br>Standard: 0.1 mg/mL<br>High: 1 mg/mL<br>Can be given via endotracheal tube | **Indications**<br>• Bolus IV therapy<br>  – Treatment of pulseless arrest<br>  – Treatment of symptomatic bradycardia unresponsive to $O_2$ and ventilation<br>• Continuous IV infusion<br>  – Shock (poor perfusion) or hypotension in patient with adequate intravascular volume and stable rhythm<br>  – Clinically significant bradycardia<br>  – β-Blocker or calcium channel blocker overdose<br>• IM bolus therapy<br>  – Pulseless arrest when bolus therapy fails.<br>  – Anaphylaxis<br>  – Severe status asthmaticus<br><br>**Precautions**<br>• May produce tachyarrhythmias<br>• High-dose infusions may produce vasoconstriction or may compromise perfusion; low doses may decrease renal and splanchnic blood flow<br>• Do not mix with sodium bicarbonate<br>• Correct hypoxemia<br>• Contraindicated in treatment of VT secondary to cocaine (may be considered if VF develops) | **Pulseless Arrest**<br>• **IV/IO dose:** 0.01 mg/kg (0.1 mL/kg of the 0.1 mg/mL concentration)<br>  – Administer every 3-5 minutes during arrest (maximum dose: 1 mg)<br>• **All endotracheal doses:** 0.1 mg/kg (0.1 mL/kg of the 1 mg/mL concentration). Administer every 3-5 minutes of arrest until IV/IO access achieved; then begin with first IV dose<br><br>**Symptomatic Bradycardia**<br>• **All IV/IO doses:** 0.01 mg/kg (0.1 mL/kg of the 0.1 mg/mL concentration)<br>• **All endotracheal doses:** 0.1 mg/kg (0.1 mL/kg of the 1 mg/mL concentration)<br><br>**Continuous IV/IO Infusion**<br>Once tubing is primed, titrate to response: typical initial infusion: 0.1-1 mcg/kg per minute; higher doses may be effective<br><br>**Anaphylaxis/Severe Status Asthmaticus**<br>• **IM dose:** 0.01 mL/kg (0.01 mg/kg of the 1 mg/mL concentration)<br>  – Maximum single dose: 0.3 mg<br>• Repeat as needed |

## Etomidate

### Indications

- Ultrashort-acting nonbarbiturate, nonbenzodiazepine sedative-hypnotic agent with no analgesic properties
- Produces rapid sedation with minimal cardiovascular or respiratory depression
- Sedative of choice for hypotensive patients
- Decreases ICP, cerebral blood flow, and cerebral basal metabolic rate

### Precautions

- May suppress cortisol production after a single dose; consider administration of stress dose hydrocortisone (2 mg/kg; maximum dose 100 mg)
- Avoid routine use in septic shock
- May also cause myoclonic activity (coughing, hiccups) and may exacerbate focal seizure disorders
- Relative contraindications include known adrenal insufficiency or history of focal seizure disorder

### For Rapid Sedation

- IV/IO dose of 0.2-0.4 mg/kg infused over 30-60 seconds will produce rapid sedation that lasts 10-15 minutes
- Maximum dose: 20 mg

| Drug/Therapy | Indications/Precautions | Pediatric Dosage |
| --- | --- | --- |
| **Glucose** | **Indications**<br>Treatment of hypoglycemia (documented or strongly suspected)<br><br>**Precautions**<br>• Use bedside glucose test to confirm hypoglycemia; hyperglycemia may worsen neurologic outcome of cardiopulmonary arrest or trauma; do not administer routinely during resuscitation<br>• Maximum concentration for newborn administration: 12.5% (0.125 g/mL) | **IV/IO Infusion**<br>• 0.5-1 g/kg (maximum recommended IV/IO concentration: 25%; can prepare by mixing 50% dextrose 1:1 with sterile water)<br>  – **50%** dextrose (0.5 g/mL): give 1-2 mL/kg<br>  – **25%** dextrose (0.25 g/mL): give 2-4 mL/kg<br>  – **10%** dextrose (0.1 g/mL): give 5-10 mL/kg<br>  – **5%** dextrose (0.05 g/mL): give 10-20 mL/kg if volume tolerated |
| **Ipratropium Bromide** | **Indications**<br>Anticholinergic and bronchodilator used for treatment of asthma<br><br>**Precautions**<br>May cause pupil dilation if it enters eyes | **Inhalation Dose**<br>250-500 mcg (by nebulizer, MDI) every 20 minutes × 3 doses |

## Lidocaine

Can be given via endotracheal tube

### Indications
- Bolus therapy
  - VF/pulseless VT
  - Wide-complex tachycardia (with pulses)
- RSI: May decrease ICP response during laryngoscopy

### Precautions/Contraindications
- High plasma concentration may cause myocardial and circulatory depression, possible CNS symptoms (eg, seizures)
- Reduce infusion dose if severe CHF or low cardiac output is compromising hepatic and renal blood flow
- Contraindicated for bradycardia with wide-complex ventricular escape beats

**VF/Pulseless VT**
- **IV/IO**
  - Initial: 1 mg/kg IV/IO loading dose
  - Maintenance: 20-50 mcg/kg per minute IV/IO infusion (repeat bolus dose if infusion initiated >15 minutes after initial bolus therapy)
- **Endotracheal**: 2-3 mg/kg

**RSI**
1-2 mg/kg IV/IO

---

## Magnesium Sulfate

50% = 500 mg/mL

### Indications
- Torsades de pointes or suspected hypomagnesemia
- Status asthmaticus not responsive to β-adrenergic drugs

### Precautions/Contraindications
- Contraindicated in renal failure
- Possible hypotension and bradycardia with rapid bolus

**Pulseless VT With Torsades**
25-50 mg/kg IV/IO bolus
(maximum dose: 2 g)

**Torsades (With Pulses), Hypomagnesemia**
25-50 mg/kg IV/IO
(maximum dose: 2 g) over 10-20 minutes

**Status Asthmaticus**
25-50 mg/kg IV/IO
(maximum dose: 2 g) over 15-30 minutes

# Pediatric Advanced Life Support Drugs

| Drug/Therapy | Indications/Precautions | Pediatric Dosage |
|---|---|---|
| **Milrinone**<br><br>Can be given IV/IO/IM/ subcutaneously | **Indications**<br>Cardiogenic shock or heart failure marked by low contractility, high vascular resistance, or both<br><br>**Precautions/Contraindications**<br>• May cause hypotension (particularly with loading dose)<br>• May cause arrhythmias<br>• Eliminated by renal excretion; use with caution in patients with renal insufficiency<br>• Avoid in patients with ventricular outflow tract obstruction | **Loading Dose (not always indicated or appropriate, due to hypotension potential)**<br>50 mcg/kg; administer over 10-60 minutes; monitor for hypotension<br><br>**IV infusion**<br>Maintenance dose (continuous IV infusion): 0.25-0.75 mcg/kg per minute |
| **Naloxone**<br><br>Can be given IV/IO/IM/ subcutaneously<br><br>Can be given via endotracheal tube; other routes preferred | **Indications**<br>To reverse effects of narcotic toxicity: respiratory depression, hypotension, and hypoperfusion<br><br>**Precautions**<br>• Half-life of naloxone often shorter than half-life of narcotic: repeated dosing is often required<br>• Administration to infants of addicted mothers may precipitate seizures or other withdrawal symptoms<br>• Assist ventilation before administration to avoid sympathetic stimulation<br>• May reverse effects of analgesics; consider administration of nonopioid analgesics for treatment of pain | **Bolus IV/IO/IM/ Subcutaneous Dose**<br>For total reversal of narcotic effects, give 0.1 mg/kg every 2 minutes PRN (maximum dose: 2 mg)<br><br>*Note:* If total reversal is not required (eg, respiratory depression), smaller doses (0.001-0.005 mg/kg [1-5 mcg/kg]) may be used. Titrate to effect.<br><br>**Continuous IV/IO infusion**<br>0.002-0.16 mg/kg (2-160 mcg/kg) per hour IV/IO infusion |

## Nitroglycerin

**Indications**
- Heart failure (especially associated with myocardial ischemia)
- Hypertensive emergency
- Pulmonary hypertension

**Precautions**
May cause hypotension, especially in hypovolemic patients

**Dose (Continuous IV Infusion)**
- Initial dose: 0.25-0.5 mcg/kg per minute
- Titrate by 1 mcg/kg per minute every 15-20 minutes as tolerated
- Typical dose range: 1-5 mcg/kg per minute (maximum dose: 10 mcg/kg per minute)
- In adolescents, start with 5-10 mcg per minute (this dose is not per kilogram per minute), and increase to maximum of 200 mcg per minute

## Nitroprusside
(Sodium nitroprusside)

Mix in $D_5W$

Vasodilator that reduces tone in all vascular beds

**Indications**
- Shock or low cardiac output states (cardiogenic shock) characterized by high vascular resistance
- Severe hypertension

**Precautions**
- May cause hypotension, particularly with hypovolemia
- Metabolized by endothelial cells to cyanide, then metabolized in liver to thiocyanate and excreted by kidneys; thiocyanate and cyanide toxicity may result if administered at high rates or with decreased hepatic or renal function; monitor thiocyanate levels in patients receiving prolonged infusion, particularly if rate >2 mcg/kg per minute
- Signs of thiocyanate toxicity include seizures, nausea, vomiting, metabolic acidosis, and abdominal cramps

**IV/IO Infusion**
- 0.3-1 mcg/kg per minute initially; then titrate up to 8 mcg/kg per minute as needed
- Light sensitive; cover drug reservoir with opaque material, or use specialized administration set
- Typically change solution every 24 hours

| Drug/Therapy | Indications/Precautions | Pediatric Dosage |
|---|---|---|
| **Norepinephrine** | Sympathetic neurotransmitter with inotropic effects; activates myocardial β-adrenergic receptors and vascular α-adrenergic receptors<br><br>**Indications**<br>Treatment of shock and hypotension characterized by low systemic vascular resistance and unresponsive to fluid resuscitation<br><br>**Precautions**<br>• May produce hypertension, organ ischemia, and arrhythmias; extravasation may cause tissue necrosis (treat with phentolamine)<br>• Do not administer in same IV tubing with alkaline solutions | **IV Administration (Only Route)**<br>Begin at a rate of 0.05-0.1 mcg/kg per minute; adjust infusion rate to achieve desired change in blood pressure and systemic perfusion; max infusion rate 2 mcg/kg per minute |

## Oxygen

**Indications**
- Should be administered during stabilization of all seriously ill or injured patients with respiratory insufficiency, shock, or trauma, even if oxyhemoglobin saturation is normal
- May monitor pulse oximetry to evaluate oxygenation and titrate therapy once child has adequate perfusion

- Administer in highest possible concentration during initial evaluation and stabilization
- A nonrebreathing mask with reservoir delivers 95% oxygen with flow rate of 10-15 L/min
- After cardiac arrest, maintain oxyhemoglobin saturation 94%-99% (or as appropriate to the patient's condition) to minimize risk of oxidative injury

## Prostaglandin E₁ (PGE₁) (Alprostadil)

**Indications**
To maintain patency of ductus arteriosus in newborns with cyanotic congenital heart disease and ductal-dependent pulmonary or systemic blood flow

**Precautions**
- May produce vasodilation, hypotension, apnea, hyperpyrexia, agitation, seizures
- May produce hypoglycemia, hypocalcemia

**IV/IO Administration**
- **Initial:** 0.05-0.1 mcg/kg per minute IV/IO infusion
- **Maintenance:** 0.01-0.05 mcg/kg per minute IV/IO infusion

| Drug/Therapy | Indications/Precautions | Pediatric Dosage |
|---|---|---|
| **Sodium Bicarbonate**<br>8.4%: 1 mEq/mL in 10- or 50-mL syringe<br><br>4.2%: 0.5 mEq/mL in 10-mL syringe | **Indications**<br>• Treatment of severe metabolic acidosis (documented or following prolonged arrest) unresponsive to ventilation and oxygenation<br>• Treatment of the following:<br>  – Hyperkalemia<br>  – Sodium channel blocker toxicity, such as tricyclic antidepressants (after support of adequate airway and ventilation)<br><br>**Precautions**<br>• Routine administration is not recommended in cardiac arrest<br>• Infuse slowly<br>• Buffering action will produce carbon dioxide, so ventilation must be adequate<br>• Do not mix with any resuscitation drugs; flush IV tubing with NS before and after drug administration<br>• Infiltration will cause tissue irritation | **IV/IO Administration**<br>**Metabolic Acidosis (Severe), Hyperkalemia**<br>• IV/IO: 1 mEq/kg slow bolus<br>• 4.2% concentration recommended for use in infants <1 month of age<br><br>**Sodium Channel Blocker Overdose (eg, Tricyclic Antidepressant)**<br>1-2 mEq/kg IV/IO bolus until serum pH is >7.45 (7.50-7.55 for severe poisoning) followed by IV/IO infusion of 150 mEq $NaHCO_3$/L solution to maintain alkalosis |
| **Vasopressin** | **Indications**<br>Catecholamine-resistant hypotension<br><br>**Precautions**<br>Use with caution in patients with renal insufficiency or | Hypotension (continuous IV infusion): 0.0002-0.002 unit/kg per minute (0.2-2 milliunits/kg per minute) |